Motor Proteins
and
Molecular Motors

Motor Proteins
and
Molecular Motors

Anatoly B. Kolomeisky
Rice University, Houston, Texas

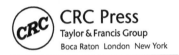

CRC Press
Taylor & Francis Group
Boca Raton London New York

CRC Press is an imprint of the
Taylor & Francis Group, an **informa** business

CRC Press
Taylor & Francis Group
6000 Broken Sound Parkway NW, Suite 300
Boca Raton, FL 33487-2742

First issued in paperback 2020

© 2015 by Taylor & Francis Group, LLC
CRC Press is an imprint of Taylor & Francis Group, an Informa business

No claim to original U.S. Government works

ISBN 13: 978-0-367-57576-2 (pbk)
ISBN 13: 978-1-4822-2475-7 (hbk)

Library of Congress Cataloging-in-Publication Data

Kolomeisky, Anatoly B., 1967- author.
  Motor proteins and molecular motors / Anatoly B. Kolomeisky.
     pages cm
  Includes bibliographical references and index.
    ISBN 978-1-4822-2475-7 (hardcover : alk. paper) 1. Biophysics. I. Title.

QH505.K65 2015
571.4--dc23

2015014853

Visit the Taylor & Francis Web site at
http://www.taylorandfrancis.com

and the CRC Press Web site at
http://www.crcpress.com

*To my daughter Ksenia
and my wife Maria*

Contents

List of Figures

List of Tables

Preface

Life is a motion! This is true at all levels of living systems, from cells to organisms, but in most cases we still do not fully understand the fundamental origin of such dynamics. In this book we would like to explore and discuss mechanisms of cellular functioning associated with several specific enzymatic molecules that are called motor proteins.

Motor proteins, also known as molecular motors, play important roles in living systems by supporting cellular transport and force generation via transformation of chemical energy into mechanical work. Examples include gene replication and transcription, protein synthesis and degradation, muscle contraction, signal transduction, transport of proteins, vesicles and organelles, cell motility, and segregation of chromosomes during cell division. Significant research activities have been undertaken in order to understand molecular mechanisms of motor protein motility and functioning. Furthermore, these efforts are also stimulated by the technological and medical needs of developing new drugs, nanoscale devices, and materials that would lead to desirable biochemical and biophysical properties of biological molecular motors. Because of the strong interdisciplinary nature of motor proteins, this research area has attracted a large and diverse set of scientists from various fields ranging from cell biology, biochemistry and biophysics to physics, materials science, and bioengineering. This field also strongly requires a unified molecular picture for analyzing motor proteins.

The central idea associated with motor protein functioning is the concept of transformation of one type of energy (chemical) into another one (mechanical). This is further complicated by the fact that molecular motors operate in solutions at isothermal but highly non-equilibrium conditions; their dynamics is coupled with multiple biochemical transitions. In addition, motor proteins move along cytoskeleton protein filaments or nucleic acid molecules in a crowded and confined cellular environment, involving a variety of chemical, mechanical, electrostatic, and hydrodynamic interactions. Taking all these factors into account in explaining the complex behavior of motor proteins is not an easy task! To develop a unified microscopic approach for analyzing complex processes in molecular motors, an application of fundamental concepts from physics and chemistry is required.

With this goal in mind, in this book we present a summary of established results, theoretical methods, and experimental observations related to biological molecular motors. In our approach we utilize fundamental physical-chemical ideas and methods in order to develop a systematic theoretical framework for understanding motor protein dynamics. The main ideas and concepts are presented using simple arguments that avoid heavy mathematical derivations in favor of more intuitive physical understanding. Although the book assumes some rudimentary knowledge of cell biology, calculus, and basic ideas from chemistry and physics, for most presented results, explanations and derivations are given. It is important to note that the book is not a comprehensive review of all known experimental and theoretical results on motor proteins. We aim here to connect major experimental facts on molecular motors to principal theoretical concepts that are consistent with the fundamental laws of chemistry and physics. It is our intention to produce a book on motor proteins that will be accessible to undergraduate, graduate students, and other researchers from a wide range of scientific fields including biology, biochemistry, biophysics, chemistry, physics, materials science, and engineering.

Acknowledgments

This book would not have been possible without my interactions and collaborations with many people over the last 20 years. I would like to thank all of them for their valuable support and intellectual discussions that stimulated my work. I especially thank Ben Widom, who introduced me to the field of motor proteins and molecular motors in 1997. The support that he kindly provided to me over many years, which also includes valuable comments on this book, are highly appreciated. I am also grateful to Michael Fisher. The close interaction with him, which continues today, was critical for my understanding of the subject. He was the one who taught me that fundamental concepts of physics and chemistry must be employed for analyzing motor proteins and molecular motors. I learned from him how to investigate complex phenomena, and how to connect theory with experiments. In addition, I wish to thank him for very careful and very critical reading of the book with multiple comments and useful suggestions that significantly improved the final version.

Over the years, I worked with many students and postdoctoral research associates on various aspects of motor proteins and molecular motors. I learned a lot from them and many ideas and methods in the book are due to their valuable contributions. I specifically thank Alexey Akimov, Max Artyomov, Rahul Das, Maria Kochugaeva, Martin Lange, Xin Li, Alex Morozov, Ekaterina Pronina, Eugene Stukalin, Hamid Teimouri, Kostas Tsekouras, Karthik Uppulury, and Alex Veksler. The help of Xin Li in preparing figures and critical reading and discussion of the book is particularly acknowledged.

My special thanks go to my friend Stas Shvartsman. He persuaded me to start this project and his constant encouragement was of great assistance to me. I am also very much indebted to my friends and experimental collaborators Michael Diehl and Peter Vekilov. Our scientific discussions greatly stimulated my work. I also thank both of them for valuable comments on this book. I benefited from discussions with many of my colleagues and friends at Rice University. I am indebted to Bob Curl, Matteo Pasquali, Peter Wolynes, Jose Onuchic, Cecilia Clementi, Marc Robert, Jim Tour, Christy Landes, and Stephan Link. But especially, I am thankful to my friend Jim Kinsey who was the first reader of the book, and who encouraged me to proceed. I am deeply grateful to him for his kind assistance over many years.

This book would not have been accomplished without long-term funding support from the National Institutes of Health, the National Science Foundation, the Welch Foundation, and the Center for Theoretical Biological Physics at Rice University. I am also thankful to many collaborators and friends outside of Rice University. In particular, the support and the tremendous encouragement from Frank Brown, Tom Chou, Debashish Chowdhury, Erwin Frey, Udo Seifert, Vladimir Gelfand, Rui Jiang, Jane Kondev, David Lacoste, Jung-Chi Liao, Martin Linden, Amit Meller, Dima Makarov, Rob Phillips, Dev Thirumalai, Andrew Spakowitz, and Sean Sun are greatly appreciated. I would like to especially thank Hong Qian for multiple stimulating discussions on fundamental issues associated with motor proteins and molecular motors. I also thank my brother, Eugene Kolomeisky, for stimulating my interest in science and for helping me over many years on various problems. His comments on this book are also very much appreciated.

Finally, it is a great pleasure to thank Francesca McGowan for her invitation to write a book on motor proteins and molecular motors and her constant encouragement throughout the writing process. I also thank Sarfraz Khan for help with the preparation and production of this book.

Author

Anatoly B. Kolomeisky is professor of chemistry and professor of chemical and biomolecular engineering at Rice University in Houston, Texas. He earned his undergraduate degree in chemistry at Moscow State University in Russia before moving to the United States in the early 1990s. He then studied physical chemistry at Cornell University with Professor Ben Widom. This was followed by postdoctoral research at the University of Maryland at College Park with Professor Michael E. Fisher. He started his independent career at Rice University in 2000. He has taught theoretical and biophysical chemistry for more than 15 years. His research interests cover a wide range of fundamental problems in physical chemistry, statistical mechanics, and biophysics, including basic mechanisms of motor proteins, thermodynamics of electrolytes, polymer translocation, artificial molecular motors and rotors, cytoskeleton dynamics, biological signaling, molecular transport through channels, biocrystallization, and protein–DNA interactions.

Professor Kolomeisky received the Camille and Henry Dreyfus New Faculty Award, the Alfred P. Sloan fellowship, and the Humboldt research fellowship.

CHAPTER 1

Introduction

CONTENTS

1.1   MOTOR PROTEINS IN BIOLOGICAL SYSTEMS

The biological cell is a main building block of all living systems. If we could take a look inside the cell (see Fig. 1.1), we would find a very complex dynamic system filled with a solution (called cytosol) of various chemical species (proteins, nucleic acids, lipids, ions, small organic molecules, etc.) and cross-linked by polymeric filamentous structures (called cytoskeleton). It would also show multiple separate compartments, a large number of spatially and temporally varying chemical reactions, significant fluxes of molecules and other particles (vesicles and organelles) between different regions of the cell, and dynamically changing cytoskeleton and cellular boundaries (Lodish et al. 2007, Alberts et al. 2007, Bray 2001)[95, 4, 23]. If we wait longer, we would witness the amazing process of cell division when a new cell, identical to the original one, is created. These complex dynamic phenomena bring to mind a suggestion (although still not quite perfect) that the biological cell is very similar in many aspects to a large city with its highly energetic life (see Fig. 1.2). As in a large city, the biological cell has different districts (compartments), cellular materials are moved in different directions mostly along specific routes, cytoskeleton filaments (roads and streets) constantly grow and shrink, and the position of cell borders is varying.

    These observations raise a fundamental question on how such complex systems as biological cells can successfully function over long periods of time in a dynamically fluctuating environment. The answer is based on the cell's unique ability to provide an adequate supply of various chemical molecules and cellular materials at localized regions when they are needed, underlying the critical importance of transport processes. For example, RNA molecules are generated in the central part of the cell, known as the nucleus (see the

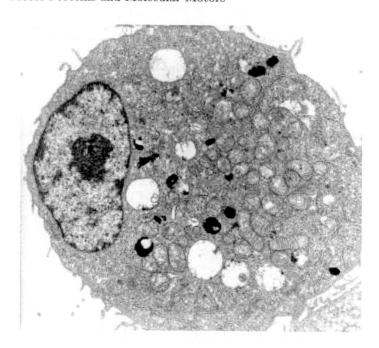

FIGURE 1.1 Transmission electron micrograph of a typical animal cell (magnified 13000 times). Various cellular structures, including nucleus (large dark oval region on the left side of the cell), mitochondria, and other organelles, are clearly seen. Adapted with permission from D. Romero et al. *Toxicology in Vitro* 17: 293–299, 2003.

large dark compartment on the left side of the cell in Fig. 1.1), but specific complexes (called ribosomes) that use them for synthesizing proteins are distributed all over the cell, so moving RNA molecules out of the nucleus is required. A major role in cellular transport is played by several classes of active enzymatic molecules called *motor proteins* (also known as biological *molecular motors*) that carry cellular materials along cytoskeleton filaments in a directed fashion. Again using a comparison with a large city (Fig. 1.2), motor proteins behave like cars and trucks that move people and materials in specific directions in the city, while the cytoskeleton filaments in the cell are playing the role of highways and streets that facilitate transport. This analogy is quite useful since it stresses some important properties of molecular motors such as directionality, efficiency, flexibility, and the ability to develop and exert forces at specific times and locations in order to overcome possible traffic jams due to molecular crowding in the cell.

Although the analogy with a large city is very useful for understanding the role of motor proteins in cellular transport, it is not exact since all particles inside the cell are in the solution, and at room temperatures each of them experiences multiple collisions with solvent molecules and with many other

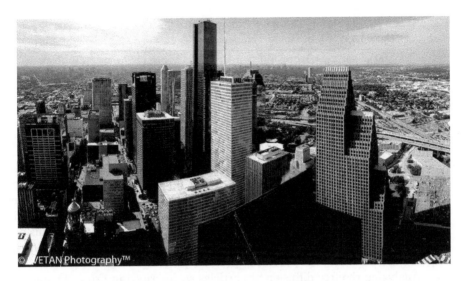

FIGURE 1.2 The view of the Houston as an example of the large city with extended network of streets and highways. The biological cells have similar complex structure.

chemical species present in the cytosol. As a result, each particle may randomly move around in the process known as a Brownian motion or diffusion that is characterized by a diffusion constant D. One might then ask the question, " why do cells need a complex cytoskeleton network and motor proteins if every particle constantly moves around and should eventually reach all possible locations in the cell?" The answer is that most cellular processes are quite fast, while unbiased diffusion (i.e., motion without a preferred direction) in most cases is slow.

To illustrate this, let us do some simple calculations. The time t to diffuse a distance r can be estimated from a simple expression,

$$t \simeq \frac{r^2}{D}. \tag{1.1}$$

(We will discuss how to derive this result in Chapter 6). The estimated average times for different particles to diffuse in water at room temperature are collected in Table 1.1. The cytosol is not water, but as a first approximation we might assume that its properties are close to pure water. Typical sizes of biological cells range from 1 μm up to 100 μm (Lodish et al. 2007, Alberts et al. 2007)[95, 4]. Small molecules and ions, which have sizes of $\simeq 0.1$ nm, can travel intracellular distances quite fast, in less than 10 s, while for protein molecules that are larger ($\simeq 1$nm) the time to diffuse across the cell is usually less than a few minutes. However, for larger organelles ($\simeq 1\mu$m) the diffusion time to move distances on the order of 100 μm is very large—close to 1 day! There are highly elongated biological cells, such as neurons, that have length

TABLE 1.1   Diffusion Times for Different Particles to Explore Specific
Distances in Water at Room Temperature

Particles	Diffusion Constant, m^2/s	Average Times to Diffuse		
		1 μm	100 μm	10 mm
Small molecules	$\simeq 10^{-9}$	$\simeq 10^{-3}$ s	$\simeq 10$ s	$\simeq 10^5$ s
Proteins	$\simeq 10^{-10}$	$\simeq 10^{-2}$ s	$\simeq 100$ s	$\simeq 10^6$ s
Organelles	$\simeq 10^{-13}$	$\simeq 10$ s	$\simeq 10^5$ s	$\simeq 10^9$ s

exceeding several centimeters and even reaching meters, and it would take many days for proteins and many years for organelles to diffuse such large distances. In addition, the mobility of large particles in the cytosol (larger than $\simeq 100$ nm) is significantly diminished due to the cytoskeleton protein filaments that create a mesh network impenetrable for organelles. Thus, we conclude that transport of large particles in cells is not possible without the special assistance that is provided by motor proteins.

Analyzing the free diffusion of particles as described in Eq. (1.1), one can note that the distance to move is proportional to the *square root* of the time ($r \propto \sqrt{t}$), and this is the main physical reason for inefficiency of unbiased diffusion in exploration of large distances. The particle returns many times to the visited site before moving into new regions. From this point of view, unbiased diffusion is inefficient in exploring new regions. In contrast, for motor proteins the traveled distances are *linearly* proportional to the time, allowing for faster delivery of cellular commodities at large distances and better exploration of new areas. The difference between these two modes of diffusion, unbiased and driven, will be discussed in detail in Chapter 6. But the advantage of employing molecular motors for transport comes with a price. They must consume energy to go so fast. Motor proteins are enzymatic molecules, which means that they accelerate various chemical reactions, and part of the energy released in these reactions is captured by molecular motors to perform their own function. Typical biochemical processes that provide energy to motor proteins include the hydrolysis of ATP (adenosine triphosphate), which is the main energy source in cellular systems (Lodish et al. 2007, Alberts et al. 2007)[95, 4], or related compounds. In addition, biological molecular motors might utilize the energy of chemical synthesis of creating main biological molecules such as DNA, RNA, and other proteins.

The transport of cellular cargoes is an important function of motor proteins, but it is not their only task. Molecular motors participate in a variety of cellular activities supporting a large number of biochemical and biophysical processes (Lodish et al. 2007, Alberts et al. 2007, Bray 2001)[95, 4, 23]. They include copying and transfer of genetic information, synthesis of relevant biological molecules (DNA, RNA and proteins), organization of cellular structures, muscle functioning, cell motility (i.e., the cell motion in the biological environment), signaling, cell division, and many others. Motor proteins are essentially involved in all processes that require mechanical work or force generation, which is critical for a large majority of cellular phenomena. Some of these processes are discussed in this book. From this point of view, one can say that the activity of molecular motors is an example of *mechanochemical coupling* since chemical energy is converted into the mechanical work. The importance of motor proteins for biological systems becomes evident when their malfunctioning leads to a variety of serious problems that include neurodegenerative disorders, Alzheimer's disease, various kidney diseases, chronic infections of the respiratory tract, myopathies (muscle diseases), and deafness (Mandelkow and Mandelkow 2002) [105].

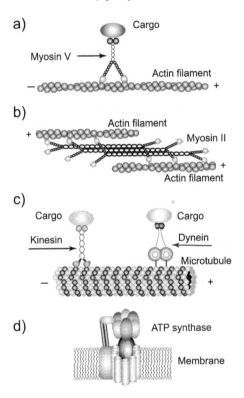

FIGURE 1.3 Schematic picture of various classes of biological molecular motors: (a) Myosin-V motor proteins that translocate the cellular cargo along actin filaments. (b) A group of myosin-II motor proteins, which also move along actin filaments, is a central component of muscles. (c) Kinesin and dynein motor proteins that transport cellular particles in opposite directions along microtubules. "Plus" and "minus" indicate that two ends of the microtubules are not the same. (d) A rotary motor protein ATP synthase.

There are many different types of molecular motors that exist in various biological systems (Lodish et al. 2007, Alberts et al. 2007, Bray 2001, Vale 2003)[95, 4, 23, 172]. Some of them are shown in Fig 1.3. The first class of motor proteins was discovered in 1940s during investigations of muscle (Banga and Szent-Gyorgyi 1942, Lodish et al. 2007, Alberts et al. 2007, Howard 2001, Pollard and Korn 1973)[95, 4, 68, 125, 15]; for this reason, this class was called myosins (from Greek "myo" for muscle)—see Fig. 1.3b. It was later realized that myosins form a large superfamily of motor proteins with a wide range of biological functions, including cellular transport and signaling (Sweeney and Houdusse 2010)[161]. Another class of molecular motors, known as dyneins, were first reported in the 1960s (Gibbons and Rowe 1965, Kardon and Vale 2009)[60, 78]. What is surprising is the fact that the most experimentally investigated motor proteins, the kinesins, were fully purified and analyzed only in 1985 (Brady 1985, Spudich et al. 1985, Vale et al. 1985)[22, 153, 173]. Dyneins and kinesins both actively participate in cellular transport and cell motility (Lodish et al. 2007, Alberts et al. 2007)[95, 4], as illustrated in Fig. 1.3c. An interesting example of the molecular motor that, in contrast to many linear motor proteins, shows rotational motion, is ATP synthase (Fig. 1.3d). These rotational motor proteins were fully analyzed only in early 1990s (Boyer 1997)[21]. Since then, many new types of molecular motors have been identified, and the list of known motor protein species is rapidly growing.

A common feature of all known motor proteins is the transformation of chemical energy into mechanical motion. It is widely believed that all motor proteins have similar mechanisms of mechanochemical coupling, although microscopic details of the process are still not well understood. There are many questions related to the fundamental principles of motor proteins operations. How is chemical energy converted into mechanical work at an atomistic level? Are there one or many mechanisms of energy transduction in molecular motors? How efficient are these processes and why? What factors determine speeds and forces produced by motor proteins? Are motor protein dynamic properties optimized or not? And if yes, what are the optimization factors: speed, force, dispersion, or something else? How molecular motors interact with each and with other cellular components, such as cytoskeleton filaments, organelles, and membranes? In this book we discuss some of these important problems from the physical-chemical point of view, underlying the connections between fundamental theoretical concepts and experimental observations.

1.2   SINGLE-MOLECULE EXPERIMENTS

The experimental method is our main tool for uncovering the mechanisms, structures, and functions of motor proteins. There are several complementary approaches that are employed for characterization of molecular motors. First, bulk chemical kinetic methods have measured rates for various transitions between biochemical states and conformations associated with the motor proteins activities (De La Cruz and Ostap 2004)[38]. Structural methods, including x-ray crystallography and cryomicroscopy, have identified the spatial arrangements of atoms and groups in various molecular conformations of motor proteins (Howard 2001, Sweeney and Houdusse 2010, Rice et al. 1999)[68, 161, 132]. But the biggest advancement in our understanding of molecular motors, especially their dynamic properties, came with the development of single-molecule techniques in the last 20 years (Howard 2001, Veigel and Schmidt 2011, Greenleaf et al. 2007)[68, 175, 63]. The application of single-molecule experimental methods have brought revolutionary changes in our views on how motor proteins function in biological systems.

There are several single-molecule methods that have been successfully applied for analyzing properties of molecular motors. Optical-trap spectroscopy, which is one of the most powerful and widely utilized methods, is based on the ability to chemically connect a single motor protein molecule to a bead that might be controlled by a calibrated external non-uniform laser field (Howard 2001, Veigel and Schmidt 2011, Greenleaf et al. 2007)[68, 175, 63]. A schematic view of experiments that use the optical-trapping systems is presented in Fig. 1.4. A related technique, known as magnetic tweezers, uses a constant magnetic field to manipulate surface-mounted single molecular motors via attached magnetic beads (Greenleaf et al. 2007)[63]. A different approach allows us to measure conformational motions of motor proteins by observing changes in resonance coupling of several fluorescent groups attached to studied molecules—the method is known as fluorescence resonance energy transfer (FRET) (Veigel and Schmidt 2011, Greenleaf et al. 2007)[175, 63]. In this case, the efficiency of energy transfer strongly depend on the distance between fluorophores. A related approach also uses fluorescence labeling for direct visualization of motor protein dynamics in solutions (Veigel and Schmidt 2011)[175]. Atomic force microscopy (AFM) is another powerful single-molecule method that provides images of molecular motors in different conformations, as well as measurements of forces exerted by these enzymes during their action (Veigel and Schmidt 2011)[175]. An important quantitative connection between cell processes and molecular dynamics of motor proteins is provided by fluorescence correlation spectroscopy methods (Weidemann et al. 2014) [180]. In this approach, a fluctuating fluorescence signal from a small detection volume in the cell is analyzed, providing important molecular and biochemical parameters of motor proteins such as concentrations, diffusion coefficients, and equilibrium constants. We will discuss multiple experimental methods and their applications for motor proteins in Chapter 3.

1.3 DISCUSSION OF THEORETICAL MODELS FOR MOLECULAR MOTORS

Intensive experimental investigations on molecular motors have allowed scientists to collect a large amount of quantitative information that stimulated a development of multiple theoretical proposals and ideas. A main goal of all theoretical methods is to understand energy transformation and coupling between biochemical reactions and mechanical motions at the microscopic level, as well as connect motor protein structures to their functions so that the

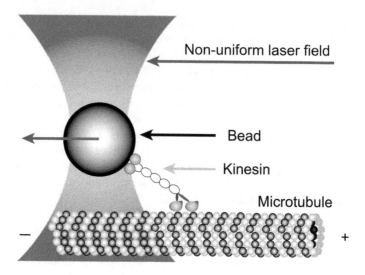

FIGURE 1.4 A simplified view of optical-trap spectroscopic experiments. A single motor protein molecule is attached to a bead that is controlled by a non-uniform laser field. Any deviations of the bead from the focus create a restoring force that influences the dynamics of the molecular motor. "Plus" and "minus" indicate that two ends of microtubules are different.

behavior of molecular motors can be successfully predicted under all conditions. But motor protein associated phenomena are very complex, so one needs to have a convenient theoretical framework in which all ideas and proposals can be successfully discussed, compared, and analyzed. It is similar to meeting a foreign person who does not speak your language, so you have to learn the foreign language, at least to some degree, in order to properly communicate. It seems that for molecular motors, such "language" should be based on physical-chemical concepts. This is due to the fact that motor proteins are catalytic molecules that speed up multiple biochemical reactions. A part of the energy released in these chemical processes is captured by molecular motors through yet unknown mechanisms and it is used for supporting various biophysical activities. The proper explanation of this mechanochemical coupling requires the use of fundamental concepts and ideas from chemistry and physics.

Adopting a physical-chemical view of motor proteins suggests that not all possible theoretical proposals could be used for understanding properties of molecular motors. We can develop a set of rules or criteria that successful theoretical models on motor proteins must satisfy:

1. Most motor proteins successfully function when they are attached to polymeric linear tracks, such as cytoskeleton protein filaments and nucleic acids. Discussing the catalytic activity of molecular motors, we typically refer

to a complex of the motor protein molecule bound to its linear track. Theoretical models must include these properties into account.

2. The activity of motor proteins is coupled to a number of chemical reactions, and it is known that all chemical processes are reversible, i.e., every reaction can go in both directions. The applicable theoretical model cannot assume irreversible transitions for explaining motor protein dynamics, even if the available experimental data might not provide strong evidence for reversibility. Experimental times are always finite, so some slow transitions might not be observed. Neglecting this might lead to serious mistakes in analysis of mechanisms for molecular motors (Kolomeisky and Fisher 2007, Kolomeisky 2013)[84, 82]. For example, not taking into account the backward rates would suggest an infinite source of energy and correspondingly infinitely large forces for motor proteins. This is clearly unphysical! We discuss this important issue in detail in Chapter 8.

3. Motor proteins are catalytic chemical molecules. It is known that catalysts accelerate *both* forward and backward chemical transitions. Theoretical models should properly reflect these enzymatic properties. More discussions on enzymatic mechanisms will be given in Chapter 5.

4. Molecular motors perform their functions in non-equilibrium systems. It means that motor protein dynamics is supported by energy input from the external sources, and when there is no energy dissipation, the net motion will not be observed (but fluctuations around the equilibrium position are always possible). The non-equilibrium nature of motor protein systems is one of the most difficult issues and it is also one of the most important properties that must be included by successful theoretical approaches. It is not possible to analyze molecular motors using only equilibrium concepts.

5. The successful model should explain existing experimental results in a quantitative manner, and it also must make experimentally testable predictions.

6. The presented theoretical ideas on molecular motors cannot violate basic laws of chemistry and physics. It seems to be a very obvious condition, but as we will see in this book there are many cases when it is forgotten.

Failure to apply these rules for critically evaluating theoretical proposals might lead to erroneous conclusions on mechanisms of molecular motors (Kolomeisky and Fisher 2007, Kolomeisky 2013, Chowdhury 2013)[84, 82, 30]. At the same time, using these physical-chemical criteria will help us to analyze current and future experimental observations for motor proteins on a strong fundamental basis.

1.4   MOTOR PROTEINS AS NANOSCALE MACHINES

A very popular view of molecular motors considers them as tiny nanoscale machines or engines that consume fuel (energy of biochemical reactions that they catalyze) in order to produce the mechanical work required by their biological functions (Howard 2001)[68]. The analogy between the biological cell and a large city gives an additional support to this view. However, one has to be careful in exploring the similarities with real machines. In reality, the working conditions for molecular motors differ significantly from the environment of macroscopic engines. Motor proteins operate at isothermal conditions at moderate temperatures in complex non-equilibrium systems, which are crowded with large quantities of chemically active biological molecules and other particles. As a result, there is a large number of random chemical and physical processes in the biological cells that might affect molecular motor dynamics. We call the systems with a strong effect from random processes *stochastic*. Despite this complexity, motor proteins are surprisingly very efficient and robust in performing their biological functions. It can be seen from the fact that any significant malfunction in motor proteins almost always leads to cell death (Lodish et al. 2007, Alberts et al. 2007, Bray 2001)[95, 4, 23]. In contrast, macroscopic engines work in deterministic conditions (where the effect of random chemical and physical processes is negligible) that also involve large temperature changes—recall the engines in our cars that burn gasoline. It is important to understand the specificity of the working environment for molecular motors in order to uncover fundamental principles that govern them.

Outstanding dynamic properties, high efficiency, and functional robustness of biological molecular motors have also stimulated significant research efforts in developing artificial molecular motors. The idea is to synthesize molecules that mimic and copy useful properties of biological molecular motors. These synthetic motors are very promising for future technological, medical, and industrial applications. But first one has to understand fundamental mechanisms of energy transformations at nanoscale. From this point of view, comparing dynamic properties of biological and artificial motors is very useful and important. In Chapter 10 we will discuss these recent developments in more detail.

1.5 OUTLOOK

As we already observed from a very brief and simplified description of molecular motors given above, their activities involve a complex network of biochemical and biophysical transformations. To disentangle connections between these processes, we argued that a physical-chemical approach should be utilized. But to understand mechanisms of motor proteins we also need to know their structural properties as well as how they are tested in various experiments. In addition, several theoretical concepts, including thermodynamics, comparison of equilibrium and non-equilibrium phenomena, random walks, and diffusion in free-energy landscapes, must be discussed in preparation for full analysis of molecular motor dynamics. It will be done in the next chapters. Then we will put all these components together in order to develop a comprehensive theoretical framework that will also allow us to understand experimental observations on molecular motors. The theoretical framework will be applied later for analyzing collective dynamics of motor proteins, which is critically important for understanding of their biological activities. At the end, artificial molecular motors and other types of biological nanoscale machines will be discussed.

More specifically, our plan for the book is the following. In Chapter 2 the history, structures, and biological functions of various motor proteins will be described. Different theoretical methods, including bulk chemical kinetic, single-molecule, and microscopy techniques, will be discussed in Chapter 3. The fundamentals of the non-equilibrium systems and its applications for molecular motors will be analyzed in Chapter 4. Chapter 5 will be devoted to explaining enzymatic properties of motor proteins. Some theoretical foundations, such as random walks, diffusion, and free-energy landscapes, will be introduced in Chapter 6. Chapter 7 will discuss theoretical analysis of motor proteins using continuum approaches. Chapter 8 will analyze theoretical discrete-state stochastic methods and their applications for explaining molecular motor dynamics. A collective dynamics of motor proteins will be discussed in Chapter 9. In Chapter 10 the artificial manmade molecular motors will be presented and analyzed. And, finally, in Chapter 11, we will present the outstanding problems associated with the motor proteins. The discussions on the future directions of the field will be also given there.

CHAPTER 2

Basic Properties of Motor Proteins

CONTENTS

2.1 HISTORY OF MOTOR PROTEINS

Since discovery of the microscope in the 17th century by Dutch tradesman-turned-scientist Antony van Leeuwenhoek (see Fig. 2.1), people started to look in great detail into phenomena that are taking place in tiny objects such as drops of water, leaves, insects, plants, soil, etc. It was realized then that processes in the microscopic world seem to be very complex and chaotic, and that biological systems are surprisingly dynamic. It was the beginning of a long quest for understanding mechanisms that generate forces and motion in living organisms. People were curious to explain these fascinating dynamic properties in cells. It became clear that the motion is closely associated with life since dead organisms do not move, although the source of this dynamic behavior was not understood.

By the mid-1900s experimental advances allowed researchers to observe many cellular processes, such as chromosome segregation and spindle dynamics during the cell division and transport of organelles to the cellular membranes. It was found that these processes include significant material fluxes and generation of strong forces. But microscopic origins of these processes could not be identified. Since in all organisms the motion is supported by muscle tissues, it was reasonable for researchers to start investigating muscles quite early, attempting to answer one the most fundamental natural question, of how movements are generated. It was a German physiologist, Wilhelm Kuhne (shown in Fig. 2.2), who in 1864 extracted from muscles a compound that he thought was a single protein responsible for the motion, so it was

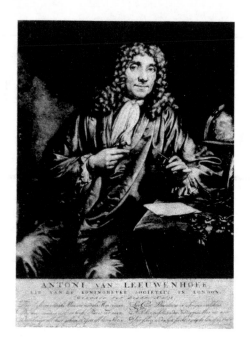

FIGURE 2.1   Antony van Leeuwenhoek (1632–1723) was a 17th century Dutch merchant who invented a powerful microscope that allowed one to observe processes in small systems. It eventually led to discovery of dynamic behavior in biological systems.

called a "myosin" (Kuhne 1864) [89]. It is interesting that Wilhelm Kuhne is also famous for introducing the term "enzyme" into the modern science language. In 1939, Russian scientists Engelhardt and Lyubimova (Engelhardt and Lyubimova 1939) [50] observed that the compound myosin could catalyze the hydrolysis of adenosine triphosphate (ATP). This was a valuable observation since it was already known that ATP is a main source of energy in biological cells (Lodish et al. 2007, Alberts et al. 2007) [95, 4]. The next important step was made in 1942 in the middle of the Second World War in the isolated Hungary by Albert Szent-Gyorgyi and his colleagues (Banga and Szent-Gyorgyi 1942) [15]. They showed that the compound extracted by Kuhne from the muscle is actually a mixture of two proteins: one of them is a motor protein, myosin, while another one is a cytoskeleton protein, actin. Albert Szent-Gyorgyi was already a famous scientist: he discovered the vitamin C, which brought him a Nobel Prize in Medicine and Physiology in 1937. In the 1950s, British scientists Hugh Huxley and Andrew Huxley (unrelated to each other) showed that both proteins could produce filaments and the muscle functioning is related to the sliding of these filaments into each other due to interactions between myosins and actin proteins (Huxley 1957, Huxley and Hanson 1954) [71, 72]. Fig. 2.4 shows the current view of how the muscles work via contraction or relaxation of actin and myosin filaments.

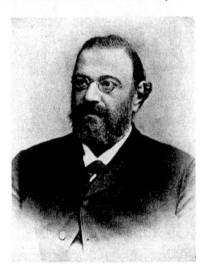

FIGURE 2.2 The German researcher Wilhelm Kuhne (1837–1900) obtained from muscle tissue a compound containing a mixture of proteins that were responsible for the functioning of the muscle.

Understanding how muscles work was a huge advance, but researchers could not repeat muscle contraction in a test tube, in so-called *in vitro* experiments, even by mixing known ingredients at cellular conditions. This problem was resolved by Jim Spudich and coworkers from Stanford University who, in 1985, developed a new experimental system which became known as a first *in vitro* motility assay (Spudich et al. 1985) [153]. It was shown that fluorescently labeled beads covered with myosin protein molecules can move directionally along properly oriented actin filaments with rates that were similar to speeds observed in real muscles. After this discovery, many other classes of myosin motors have been purified and analyzed in various cellular systems.

At the same time, it was known that highly dynamic processes can also take place in non-muscle cells. The segregation of chromosomes during cell division was the best example of such activities. The question was then: Do these dynamic processes also involve myosin motor proteins and cytoskeleton actin filaments like in muscles? The answer was negative, and it was obtained independently in 1985 by three different groups (Brady 1985, Vale et al. 1985, Scholey et al. 1985) [22, 173, 143] that observed the transport of organelles in isolated nerve cells, known as axons, of a giant squid. Surprisingly, researchers observed the motion along other cytoskeleton filaments, microtubules, so it was not myosins hopping along the actin filaments. The protein molecules responsible for the transport along microtubules have been purified, and Vale

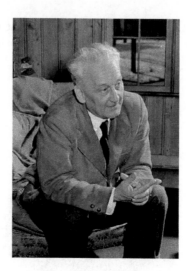

FIGURE 2.3   The Hungarian physiologist and Nobel Prize winner Albert Szent-Gyorgyi (1893–1986) who first extracted and identified myosin motor proteins from the muscles.

and colleagues (Vale et al. 1985) [173] named this enzyme "kinesin," which comes from a Greek word for motion. Since further investigations have led to discovery of a large number of species closely related to the kinesins, the original protein has been renamed as a conventional kinesin or kinesin-1.

It is known that microtubules are polar filaments, which means that the chemical structures of their ends are different (Lodish et al. 2007, Alberts et al. 2007)[95, 4], and kinesin motor proteins enable the cellular transport only in one specific direction on the microtubules, which is called the "plus" end of the microtubules. Transport in the opposite direction (to the "minus" end of the microtubules) is supported by other types of motor proteins known as dyneins. It is interesting to note that the first microtubule-based motor proteins dyneins were discovered 20 years earlier than kinesins in cellular protrusions, cilia and flagella, which are responsible for cellular locomotion and for sensing of the environment (Lodish et al. 2007, Alberts et al. 2007) [95, 4]. Strong advances in electron microscopy allowed researchers to look into these structures in great detail in the 1950s. It was found that the central part of cilia and flagella, known as the axoneme, contains pairs of microtubule filaments coupled together by unknown protein molecules. In 1965 these proteins were identified as ATPases, i.e., they could catalyze the hydrolysis of ATP, and the researchers called these proteins "dyneins," the name coming from the Greek word "dyne," or force (Gibbons and Rowe 1965) [60]. But the discovery of cytoplasmic dyneins (which function in the main body of the cell) came only in 1987 (Paschal et al. 1987, Lye et al. 1987, Roberts et al. 2013) [122, 98, 133], 2 years after finding kinesins.

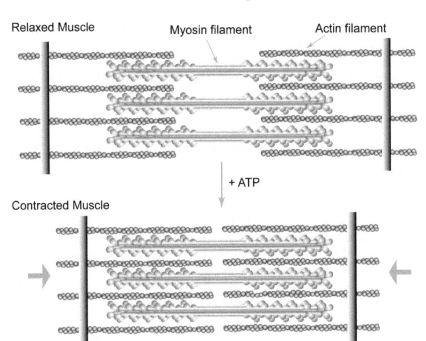

FIGURE 2.4 A schematic view of how muscles function. Filaments made from myosins and actin proteins slide into each other when ATP molecules are added, leading to muscle contraction. At low concentration of ATP the myosins unbind from the actin and filaments move away from each other, leading to muscle relaxation.

Experimental advances in many directions allowed researchers to investigate various biological processes in great detail, and it was realized that in many systems several key proteins play the role of molecular motors. For example, in 1960 several groups found that an unknown protein molecule was responsible for biosynthesis of messenger RNA molecules in the presence of DNA (Hurwitz et al. 1960, Stevens 1960) [70, 156]. This protein was called "RNA polymerase" (RNAP). But only in 2001 were Roger Kornberg and his coworkers able to obtain crystal structures of an RNA polymerase and transcription complex (Cramer et al. 2001, Gnatt et al. 2001) [36, 62]. It provided a detailed molecular view of how the RNAP molecule uses the chemical energy of RNA synthesis to advance along the DNA chain in a consistent manner while elongating the RNA chain by adding specific monomers to it. For this work that helped to explain the transcription process at the molecular level, Roger Kornberg received the Nobel Prize in Chemistry in 2006.

Employing improved experimental methods, scientists clearly showed that many other proteins, such as helicases, topoisomerases, gyrases, translocases, etc., can be viewed as biological molecular motors. Continuous efforts to describe various complex biological systems in more detail constantly led to discovery and identification of many new types of biological molecular motors. In the future, we expect to see more fascinating examples of tiny biological protein machines!

2.2 CLASSIFICATION OF BIOLOGICAL MOLECULAR MOTORS

The fact that there are many proteins that can be identified as biological motors raises a fundamental question on universality of mechanisms that govern motor proteins. However, to distinguish details of how motor proteins function at the molecular level, one needs to classify them using their physical-chemical properties. It is known that in most cases motor proteins become active enzymes only after binding to some cellular structures. These structures could be static or dynamic and they include cytoskeleton protein filaments, cellular membranes, nucleic acids, and other assemblies of biologically relevant molecules. For example, if we mix solutions containing only kinesin motor proteins, and ATP, no hydrolysis of ATP will be observed. But the hydrolysis reaction becomes fast as soon as we add a solution of microtubules. In this case kinesins quickly associate to the microtubule and then ATP molecules bind to the complex, starting the enzymatic process. Here again the analogy between cells and big cities is helpful for understanding these facts. Cars and trucks (motor proteins) can only move and perform their transport functions if roads and streets (cytoskeleton filaments) are available.

Different cellular structures that activate motor protein functioning allows us to present the following classification scheme for biological molecular motors. It is based on the chemical nature of these cellular structures (Kolomeisky 2013) [82]:

(1) *Cytoskeleton Filament Motor Proteins*: This class of molecular motors starts to work after binding and hopping along the cytoskeleton filaments, such as actin filaments or microtubules. It includes various types of kinesins, dyneins, and myosins. These motor proteins accelerate the hydrolysis of ATP molecules, and a fraction of the released chemical energy is converted into mechanical work. The cellular transport of vesicles, organelles, and other species is fully supported by these proteins. As we already discussed, the enzymatic molecules from this class were the first to be discovered, and they are also the most studied systems from the dynamic and structural points of view. Actually, most current views and explanations of energy transformations in motor proteins are based almost exclusively on the analysis of experiments from kinesins and myosin motor proteins (Howard 2001, Sweeney and Houdusse 2010, Veigel and Schmidt 2011, Kolomeisky and Fisher 2007, Kolomeisky 2013, Chowdhury 2013) [68, 161, 175, 84, 82, 30]. The cytoskeleton-bound motor proteins are illustrated in Figs. 1.2a, 1.2b, and 1.2c as well as in Fig. 2.7.

(2) *Nucleic Acid Motor Proteins*: This class of biological molecular motors includes DNA and RNA polymerases, helicases, topoisomerases, ligases, gyrases, and many other types of proteins that function by closely interacting with DNA and RNA molecules. To perform their work, nucleic acid motor proteins use the chemical energy from various processes, including polymerization and synthesis of DNA, RNA, and proteins as well as the hydrolysis of ATP or related compounds. These enzymes are critically important for cells since they are responsible for maintaining, processing, and copying of the genetic information, and for synthesis of all DNA, RNA and protein molecules in cells (Lodish et al. 2007, Alberts et al. 2007) [95, 4]. A good example to illustrate activities of nucleic acid motor proteins is presented in Fig. 2.5, where complex processes associated with DNA replication are shown. In recent years, there were significant experimental efforts devoted to measuring properties and structures of these biological motors (Cramer et al. 2001, Gnatt et al. 2001, Charvin et al. 2003, Meglio et al. 2009, Pyle 2008, Singleton et al. 2007) [36, 62, 28, 109, 126, 148]. Although we understand now much more about the functioning of nucleic acid motor proteins, their microscopic mechanisms and dynamic properties are still not well quantified and explained in many aspects, especially in comparison with the cytoskeleton motor proteins. The main reason for this is the fact that nucleic acid motor proteins participate in a variety of very complex cellular processes that involve a large number of biochemical reactions and biophysical phenomena, which are not yet well resolved. In many cases, properties of the nucleic acid motor proteins are coupled in a complex way with other biochemical processes, and these issues make it very difficult to uncover their mechanisms.

(3) *Rotary Motor Proteins*: This is a very unusual class of biological molecular motors that, in contrast to other classes that we described above, transform the chemical energy into rotational degrees of freedom (Lodish et al. 2007, Alberts et al. 2007, Berg 2003, Oster and Wang 2003, Sowa and Berry 2008, Muench et al. 2011) [95, 4, 121, 152, 115, 18]. These proteins are typically functional when bound to the cellular membranes. There are 2 types of motor proteins that are usually identified as belonging to this class. One of them is known as bacterial flagellar motors (BFM) (Sowa and Berry 2008) [152]. Most species of bacteria are able to survive by sensing the surrounding medium and moving in the direction of favorable conditions (Lodish et al. 2007, Alberts et al. 2007) [95, 4]. This motion is supported by flagella, which can be viewed as long helical filaments that extend from the cell main body, and it is driven by BFM. A typical bacterium with multiple flagella is shown in Fig. 2.6. Note that these cellular extensions might be larger in length than the cell itself! The energy source for these motors comes from the difference in ion concentrations (H^+ or Na^+) inside and outside of the cellular membrane, so these species can also be considered as electrochemical motors. These systems are one of the largest known protein machines and their functioning requires many other types of various auxiliary protein molecules (Sowa and Berry 2008). This complexity is probably the main reason that

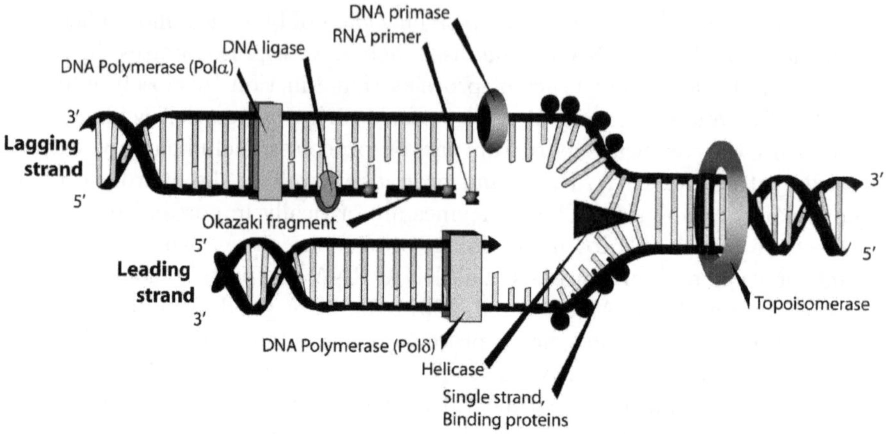

FIGURE 2.5 A simplified graphical view of DNA replication. Participating nucleic acid motor proteins are indicated. During this process identical copies of the original DNA molecule are created by the actions of several different motor proteins that are involved at different stages. The figure is adopted from Wikimedia Commons.

mechanisms of torque generation in bacterial flagella motors are still not well understood. In addition, since these proteins are membrane-bound, there are no high-resolution crystal structures available (Berg 2003, Sowa and Berry 2008) [18, 152], complicating research efforts to explore their mechanisms.

Another type of rotary molecular motor is known as rotary ATPases, and it consists of 3 membrane protein complexes (Muench et al. 2011) [115]. These motors are shown schematically in Fig. 1.2d. Each of these protein complexes has 2 different rotating motors connected together (Oster and Wang 2003, Muench et al. 2011) [121, 115]. The bacterial proteins F_1F_0-ATPase (F-ATPase), also known as ATP synthases, are reversible rotational machines. At one set of conditions they might use the ion gradients to help the synthesis of ATP molecules, while for low gradients the rotational direction is reversed and they use the hydrolysis of ATP for moving ions across the membrane. Cells from organisms more complex than bacteria (*eukaryotic* cells) have another rotary ATPase, which is known as a vacuolar H^+-ATPase (V-ATPase). In nature these proteins mostly operate as ATP-driven pumps for proton ions, while it has been shown that they also can synthesize ATP in *in vitro* conditions (Muench et al. 2011) [115]. In some bacteria and in other simple organisms called archaea there is a third member of the rotary ATPases known as A_1A_0-ATPase (A-ATPase). They are also reversible rotational engines, similar to F-ATPases, that couple ATP synthesis and ion pumping functions (Muench et al. 2011) [115]. Significant structural and dynamic information about these motors is already collected in a large number of experiments, but full understanding of energy transduction mechanisms is still not available. However,

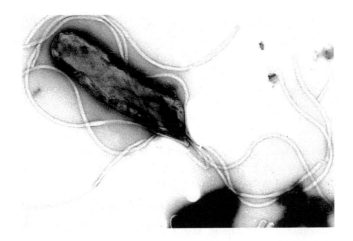

FIGURE 2.6 Electron micrograph of *H. pylori* bacteria with multiple flagella. Darker oval region is a bacterial body, while lighter extensions are flagella. Published with full permission from Prof. Y. Tsutsumi.

there are theoretical arguments (Oster and Wang 2003, Kolomeisky and Fisher 2007) [121, 84], suggesting that mechanisms of energy transformation in rotary motor proteins are probably quite similar to those of linear biological motors (such as kinesins, myosins and dyneins). So ideas developed for translocating motor proteins might also be applied for rotary motors. It remains to be fully tested in future experimental and theoretical investigations.

Concentrating more on linear motors, we notice that they can also be subdivided in two large groups. This classification scheme is based on the number of enzymatic cycles that the motor protein molecule supports during each active encounter with the cytoskeleton filaments or nucleic acids. It is also a measure of how tightly molecular motors are attached to their cellular tracks. The stronger the motor is associated with the cytoskeleton filament or nucleic acid, the more enzymatic processes can be accomplished. There are many classes of motor proteins that are strong enough to perform their duties while moving long distances along cytoskeleton filaments or nucleic acids without detachments. We know multiple examples of such motors that include kinesins and dyneins that move in opposite directions along the microtubules, myosins-V and myosins-VI that translocate in opposite directions along actin filaments, RNA and DNA polymerases that closely follow DNA molecules (but usually only in one specific direction), helicases that unwind double-stranded DNA chains, and many other motor proteins. They usually function as single species, and the way they work can be compared to the action of individual heavy tracks or railway locomotives. These motor proteins are known as *processive molecular motors*.

One could think that the processivity is a critical property that all biological molecular motors should possess. Otherwise, how could they exert forces in a consistent fashion? Surprisingly, there are many motor proteins that are *non-processive*, i.e., they typically take one or few steps along cellular tracks before dissociating. The most known example is muscle myosins (Howard 2001, Sweeney and Houdusse 2010) [68, 161]. And there are other types of motor proteins that experiments suggest are non-processive. For example, there is a kinesin motor protein Ncd that, in contrast to conventional kinesins, cannot sustain long trajectories along microtubule filaments (Endow and Barker 2003) [140]. This raises a question as to how these proteins are able to produce mechanical forces and how they function. It turned out that in all these cases non-processive motor proteins work in large groups (recall myosins in muscles). Obviously, many motors must interact with each other in order to function under these circumstances. However, although several ideas have been presented, mechanisms of this cooperativity are still not fully explained (Kolomeisky 2013)[82]. We will discuss more collective dynamics of motor proteins in Chapter 9.

If one would like to understand why some biological molecular motors are processive while others are not, experimental studies suggest that in most cases this property closely correlates with the molecular structures of proteins (Kozielski et al. 1997, Tomishige et al. 2002) [88, 100]. Non-processive motor proteins typically exist in monomeric forms, while processive motors have complex dimeric and oligomeric structures. (Howard 2001, Bray 2001) [23, 68]. Then it is clear that oligomeric motor proteins have a higher probability of staying attached to cellular structures, and that keeps them in the active state longer. This is because the probability that all track-binding domains of motor proteins will simultaneously dissociate from their tracks strongly decreases with the number of monomers in the molecule. Thus the monomer motor proteins will stay attached to the cellular structure for the shortest period of time, which leads them to be non-processive. It is interesting that these arguments should be modified for nucleic motor proteins. These motors can be viewed as heterogeneous multimeric molecules where typically only one domain is catalytically active. Other non-motor domains support the high processivity of these enzyme by being attached to nucleic acids in a "clamp-like" fashion, providing these biological motors enough time to successfully proceed and not to dissociate (Singleton et al. 2007) [148].

2.3 STRUCTURES OF MOTOR PROTEINS

All known motor protein molecules have complex multi-domain structures; see, for example, Fig. 2.7 where structures of several cytoskeleton motor proteins are shown (Alberts et al. 2007, Lodish et al. 2007, Howard 2001, Marx et al. 2005) [4, 95, 68, 107]. This is expected given the multitude of cellular tasks that they have to perform. The complexity helps molecular motors to overcome multiple barriers that exist in crowded and noisy cellular environment, and it also supports their robust functioning under dynamic conditions.

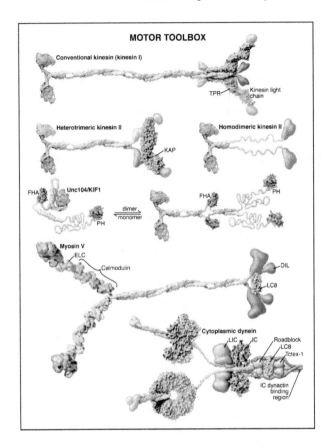

FIGURE 2.7 Multi-domain structures of various cytoskeleton motor proteins. The results are obtained from atomic resolution measurements. The figure is adopted with permission from Vale 2003 [172].

To illustrate more specifically the multi-domain nature of motor proteins, let us consider conventional kinesins which structurally are well characterized (Vale 2003, Kozielski et al. 1997, Marx et al 2005) [172, 88, 107]. This motor can be viewed as a prototypical example for many cytoskeleton motor proteins. The domain structure of the kinesin-1 molecule attached to the microtubule filament is shown in Fig. 2.8. This molecular motor binds the microtubule via so-called *motor head* or *catalytic domains*. These are the most important parts of the motor since the enzymatic reaction of ATP hydrolysis takes place here. At the other end of the molecule there is a *tail* region with two light chains; see Fig. 2.8. These domains are important for transport since they are responsible for strong binding to cellular cargoes (sometimes indirectly via associating to other molecules known as scaffolding proteins). There are other domains, such as *neck linker, neck,* and *coiled–coil stalk* that connect together catalytic and cargo-binding regions of the molecule, providing mechanical flexibility (note a *hinge* in the middle of the coiled-coil stalk region in Fig. 2.8) and chemical stability. The important note here is that the directionality of kinesin motors (to go into the plus or minus direction along the microtubules) is determined by the chemical composition of the neck domain (Endow and Barker 2003) [140]. The reason for this is still not fully understood, but one could speculate that changing the chemical composition of the neck modifies the overall interactions of the motor protein domains with the microtubule, creating effective asymmetric potentials of interactions that might have different directions. Although other cytoskeleton motor proteins might have some variations in their structures, the overall molecular plan is similar to conventional kinesins (Alberts et al. 2007, Lodish et al. 2007, Howard 2001, Marx et al. 2005) [4, 95, 68, 107]. Surprisingly, more complex domain structures are found for dynein motor proteins (see the bottom of Fig. 2.7) (Roberts et al. 20013) [133], and the reason for such complexity is still not clear.

Thinking about the structures of biological molecular motors, the analogy between them and big trucks that are driven on roads is quite useful. The catalytic domains can be viewed as the engine, the tail corresponds to the truck bed, and the other domains play roles similar to the truck frame. However, there are significant differences between motor proteins and macroscopic machines. In molecular motors, domains might strongly interact with each other, leading to modification and even inhibition of their enzymatic activities. There are several experimental observations for some kinesin and myosin motor proteins indicating that partial unfolding of cargo-binding domains might completely stop the catalytic functioning of motor domains (Liu et al. 2006, Thirumurugan et al. 2006, Dietrich et al. 2008) [94, 162, 42]. This means that our nanoscale trucks do not work when there is no load. We know that our macroscopic trucks can be driven without a load. This interesting observation suggests that the performance of biological motors might be optimized with respect to their fuel consumption so that there are not many futile processes. Apparently, the fuel is much more expensive at the cellular level as compared with our everyday life, so that biological molecular machines are much more efficient in comparison with cars that we drive!

Nucleic acid bound motor proteins also have complex multi–domain structures. For example, the molecular geometry for RNA polymerases (Pol)I obtained from crystal structures is presented in Fig. 2.9 (Engel et al. 2013) [49]. This motor protein is important in regulating the cell growth. This is because during the transcription process, which corresponds to reading genes from DNA and copying them to RNA molecules, it produces the RNA part of ribosome complexes where all proteins are synthesized. It has 14 subunits that interact with each other in a complex manner (see Fig. 2.9). Similar to cytoskeleton motor proteins, this enzyme has a subunit with the active site (domain A12.2 in Fig. 2.9). The role of other domains is to support a variety of processes including RNA chain initiation, elongation, proofreading, and termination while being attached to DNA molecules. Again we can see that

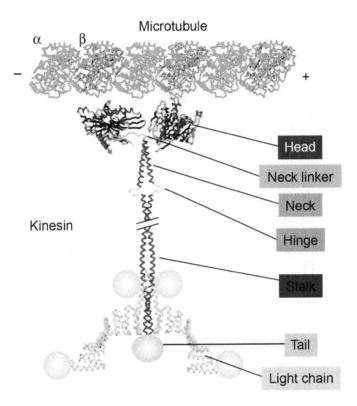

FIGURE 2.8 A diagrammatic view of various protein domains in the conventional kinesin molecule, which is attached to a microtubule filament. It is obtained by analyzing known high-resolution molecular structures. The figure is adopted with permission from Mandelkow and Mandelkow 2002 [105].

the efficient solving of multiple tasks by motor proteins requires them to have multi-domain structures.

2.4 BIOLOGICAL FUNCTIONS OF MOLECULAR MOTORS

Motor proteins are involved as key elements in a large number of biological processes where mechanical forces and torques need to be generated locally at specific times (Lodish et al. 2007, Alberts et al. 2007, Howard 2001) [95, 4, 68]. One of the main functions of biological molecular motors is transport. This is relevant mostly for cytoskeleton motor proteins such as kinesins, dyneins, and myosins that move various cellular cargoes (vesicles, organelles, virus particles, pathogens, and other cellular structures) along cytoskeleton tracks (Hirokawa et al. 2009, Vale 2003, Roberts et al. 2013) [65, 172, 133]. The importance of

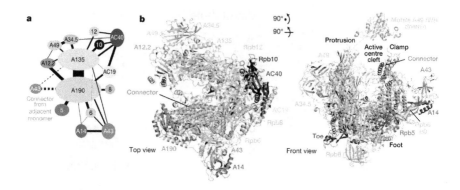

FIGURE 2.9   Crystal structure and protein domains for yeast RNA polymerase. (a) A map of different subunits and their interactions. (b) Top and side views of the protein's structure. The figure is adopted with permission from Engel et al. 2013 [49].

molecular motors for cellular transport can be seen from the fact that problems and defects in the long-distance traffic in neurons and asymmetric cells due to malfunctioning of several types of kinesin molecules have been directly associated with various neurodegenerative diseases such as Alzheimer's decease and human neuropathy (Mandelkow and Mandelkow 2002) [105]. The failure to remove large pathogen particles and viruses, which due to their large sizes can exit cells only with the help of motor proteins, can also lead to virus infections (Mandelkow and Mandelkow 2002) [105]. A related function of cytoskeleton motor proteins is a participation in the cellular signal transduction processes via transportation of proteins and other molecules that are important for signaling cascades (Hirokawa et al. 2009) [65].

Cytoskeleton motor proteins also play main roles during cell division when they help to organize and guide the necessary cellular structures such as microtubules, chromosomes, and a spindle (a cellular structure that is utilized for segregating chromosomes). In this process, biological motors directly apply forces to assemble microtubules into the spindle, to connect them to chromosomes, to move chromosomes in specific directions. Some motor proteins might also regulate the length of microtubules via association and dissociation processes because of their double roles as motors and polymerases and depolymerases (Lodish et al. 2007, Alberts et al. 2007, Howard 2001, Reese et al. 2014) [95, 4, 68, 130]. If motor proteins do not work properly during the cell division, it might lead to serious consequences such as cancer (Mandelkow and Mandelkow 2002) [105].

Nucleic acid motor proteins participate in a variety of cellular processes by assisting in maintenance, copying, and transfer of genetic information (Lodish et al. 2007, Alberts et al. 2007, Pyle 2008) [95, 4, 126], see also Fig. 2.5. Their functions include the unwinding of double-stranded DNA molecules, the recognition of different bases on DNA, copying them into RNA molecules, correcting of chemical and topological defects in DNA chains, synthesis of proteins, assisting in RNA folding, and many others.

The strongly bound to cellular membrane rotary motor proteins also have multiple biological functions. In bacterial cells the bacterial flagellar motor drives the rotation of flagella (see Fig. 2.6) which is the main mechanism of bacterial swimming and testing the environment (Berg 2003, Sowa and Berry 2008) [18, 152]. Other ATPase rotary motor proteins at some conditions (high ionic potential across cellular membranes) synthesize ATP molecules, the main source of energy in biological cells, while at less favorable conditions they utilize the hydrolysis of ATP to pump ions in order to support the membrane potential (Oster and Wang 2003, Muench et al. 2011) [121, 115]. Maintaining the membrane ionic potential is critically important for cells, to survive for long periods of time.

Furthermore, we should clearly understand that there are many other biological functions of motor proteins that we still do not know. The progress in experimental studies will definitely bring to the light new roles for biological molecular motors.

2.5 SUMMARY

In this chapter we presented a fascinating history of discoveries of different classes of motor protein species. The driving force for all these advances was the desire to understand mechanisms of force production in biological systems. Since the number and variety of biological molecular motors is so large, in order to better understand their functioning, two classification schemes, depending on their physical-chemical properties, were introduced. One is based on the chemical nature of cellular structures that activate molecular motors, while another one accounts for a persistence in supporting enzymatic cycles.

Our analysis of motor proteins started with a discussion of their molecular structures. It was argued that the complexity of biological tasks that they have to accomplish is the main reason for multi-domain structures. Other reasons include the support for mechanical flexibility and chemical stability. The important property of motor proteins is that different subunits might strongly interact with the another, probably, to optimize their performance. We analyzed and compared several specific molecular structures.

CHAPTER 3

Experimental Studies of Motor Proteins

CONTENTS

3.1   INTRODUCTION

Our knowledge of how motor proteins work comes from many different experimental sources. It is important to note that multiple experimental methods give us complementary information on various aspects of biological molecular motor functioning. Bulk biochemical kinetic studies provide an average dynamic description of relevant chemical processes associated with motor proteins, including equilibrium constants, relaxation times to stationary states, chemical reaction rates, and changes in concentrations of motor species with time (De La Cruz and Ostap 2004, Fischer et al. 2010, Gilbert and Mackey 2000) [38, 54, 61]. Structural studies allow researchers to determine spatial positions of various atoms in different molecular conformations, and they also help to choose the most relevant chemical states from the point of view of supporting dynamics of molecular motors (Howard 2001, Rice et al 1999, Sweeney and Houdusse 2010, Kozielski et al. 1997, Marx et al. 2005, Marx et al. 2009) [68, 132, 161, 88, 107, 106]. Single-molecule investigations concentrate on dynamic and mechanical properties of individual molecules during their motion on various cellular structures (Howard 2001, Veigel and Schmidt 2011, Greenleaf et al. 2007, Dulin et al. 2013) [68, 175, 63, 46]. The crucial observation is that these methods allow modifications of the activities of individual motors via applying external loads and changing rates of chemical transitions. Microscopy measurements lead to visualization of motor protein molecules in different biochemical states (Veigel and Schmidt 2011, Greenleaf et al. 2007) [175, 63]. To understand the fundamental mechanisms of motor proteins, one has to combine and utilize all information obtained by different techniques. However, a critical analysis of what these experiments actually can tell us is needed. There are drawbacks, limitations, uncertainties, and specific assumptions associated with each method, and these factors should be taken into account if we wish to fully understand how motor proteins function.

In this chapter, we discuss various experimental methods of studying motor proteins. Our goal is to clarify strong and weak sides and to understand the abilities and limitations of each experimental technique. We will analyze various experimental approaches and how information is extracted from them using simple physical-chemical arguments. It will help us to connect experimental results with theoretical ideas in following chapters.

3.2   BULK CHEMICAL-KINETIC MEASUREMENTS

The functioning of motor proteins is associated with a large number of biochemical processes such as binding and unbinding from cellular structures (cytoskeleton filaments, nucleic acids, and cellular membranes), enzymatic reactions, release of products of enzymatic processes, and many others (Lodish et al. 2007, Alberts et al. 2007, Bray 2001, Howard 2001) [95, 4, 23, 68]. These chemical reactions drive structural changes, conformational transitions, and force generation in biological molecular motors.

There are several chemical-kinetic methods to investigate enzymatic processes (Houston 2001, Gilbert and Mackey 2000, Cook and Cleland 2007) [67, 61, 33]. In most situations, one has to start with accurate measurements of protein concentrations at different times. This is typically accomplished by utilizing various spectroscopic methods (Atkins and de Paula 2009) [10]. The idea is that one can measure separately the light intensity coming into the protein solution sample (I_0) and the intensity of the light after passing the sample (I). Using these two measured quantities a new function, called *absorbance*, A, is defined,

$$A = \log \frac{I_0}{I}. \qquad (3.1)$$

The larger absorbance A, the less light is coming out of the sample. Then there is an empirical law known as the *Beer–Lambert law* (which can be also justified from some fundamental concepts) that connects the absorbance with the concentration c of dissolved protein molecules in the solution via (Atkins and de Paula 2009) [10]

$$A = \varepsilon c l, \qquad (3.2)$$

where l is the path length of the light (known in these experiments) and a proportionality coefficient ε is called the *molar absorption coefficient*. The parameter ε for motor proteins can be well estimated from the composition of amino acids (Gilbert and Mackey 2000) [61]. This is a very robust and efficient technique of measuring motor protein concentrations for not very concentrated systems and under conditions such that no other molecular associations (frequently called *oligomerizations*) are taking place. A related method uses the radioactive isotopes and their emissions to quantify concentrations of studied species (Mackey and Gilbert 2000) [101]. These methods work well for kinesin motor proteins as well as for nucleic acid processive enzymes (Fischer et al. 2010) [54]. For other cytoskeleton motor proteins, myosins, and dyneins, standard titration techniques have been also employed (Gilbert and Mackey 2000) [61].

Having several reliable methods of measuring concentrations at different times allows researchers to directly investigate kinetic properties of motor proteins. To compare enzymatic efficiency of different motor species it is convenient first to analyze the steady-state kinetics. These experiments must be performed at high saturating concentrations of cellular structures (cytoskeleton filaments, nucleic acids) and substrates (usually ATP) in order to make sure that other slower kinetic processes do not interfere (Gilbert and Mackey 2000, Fischer et al. 2010) [61, 54].

Much more mechanistic information on motor proteins can be obtained from pre-steady-state kinetic measurements (Cook and Cleland 2007, Gilbert and Mackey 2000, Fischer et al. 2010) [33, 61, 54]. These experiments provide detailed information on kinetic rates for individual chemical transitions involving molecular motors. Several methods have been developed for this type of kinetic studies, but all of them require strong mixing of components. The reason for this is that if one does not mix reactants well, the overall rate of the studied chemical reactions will be determined after some time not by the chemical processes themselves but by the diffusion of molecules. This is not a desired outcome for motor protein investigations.

There are two main approaches for investigating kinetics of motor proteins that do not reach the stationary-state conditions. One of them is known as a *Rapid Chemical Quench-Flow Method* (Gilbert and Mackey 2000, Barman et al. 2006) [61, 16]. This is a method that has a long history (more than 70 years), and it involves a rapid mixing of enzymes and substrate molecules to initiate the chemical reaction. The reaction can be terminated at specific later times by adding a quenching agent. In most cases the quenching agent is a strong acid (hydrochloric acid, formic acid, trifluoroacetic acid), although other chemical compounds such as a strong alkali, SDS (the surface-active compound), and EDTA (the compound that strongly binds to some metal ions) have also been used (Barman et al. 2006) [16]. The role of the quenching agent is to unfold all participating protein molecules, effectively stopping any enzymatic reaction. In some cases, the rapid change in temperature (so-called *temperature quench* or *physical quench*) via rapid freezing or evaporation can also produce the same results. This method allows measurement of the chemical composition of the solution at different times, providing a full description of chemical kinetic processes associated with motor proteins. The illustration of this method can be given in the example presented in Fig. 3.1 where the kinetics of kinesin Ncd motor proteins is measured by analyzing the formation of ADP (the product of ATP hydrolysis) for different initial concentrations of ATP (Foster and Gilbert 2000) [56]. One can see in Fig. 3.1A the increase in the amount of the product of the reaction (ADP) as a function of time, and these data are then fitted to a so-called *burst biphasic equation* (Foster and Gilbert 2000) [56],

$$[ADP] = A\left[1 - \exp\left(-k_b t\right)\right] + k_2 t, \tag{3.3}$$

where k_b is the rate constant of the pre-steady-state burst phase, A is the amplitude of the burst of ADP formation, and k_2 is the rate constant corresponding to the steady-state turnover. Burst rate constants and amplitudes at different initial ATP concentrations are shown in Figs. 3.1B and 3.1C, respectively.

The quench-flow method is a powerful technique that helps to identify and chemically characterize intermediates in enzymatic reaction pathways for a variety of motor proteins systems (Gilbert and Mackey 2000, Fischer et l. 2010) [61, 54]. The main advantage of the method is that it does not need to use complex optical systems. It is quite robust and versatile, and it can be easily coupled to an array of modern chemical analytical methods. However, there are also limitations in the application of the quench-flow technique. This is a chemical sampling method that requires significant time and effort in order to analyze every sample. Another weak point is the analysis of data; in many cases simplified kinetic models have been utilized without proper critical assessments. The danger here is that quite different kinetic models might lead to similar experimental observations.

Much more popular in kinetic studies of motor proteins is a *stopped-flow method* (Gilbert and Mackey 2000, Dillingham et al. 2002) [61, 43]. In this method, the investigated mixture of reactants is injected into the system and the reaction mixture is stopped in the experimental chamber — this is the reason for the name "stopped flow." This stopping also triggers data collection. The optical signal of the sample is measured and it is correlated with the temporal evolution of various chemical processes in the system. Depending on specific conditions, the optical signal could be obtained from light scattering, absorbance, fluorescence, or turbidity measurements. To explain this method let us consider a specific example of kinetic measurements of ATP-dependent translocation of a PcrA helicase motor protein along single-stranded DNA chains (Dillingham et al. 2002) [43]. The molecular motors bind to DNA and move in a specific direction. In these experiments, a fluorescent analogue of DNA base was used as a source of the optical signal. DNA molecules consist of monomers that are typically called bases or nucleotides. In this case, one fluorescent monomer was attached to the end of a non-fluorescent DNA along which the helicase was hopping. It was shown that the fluorescent intensity

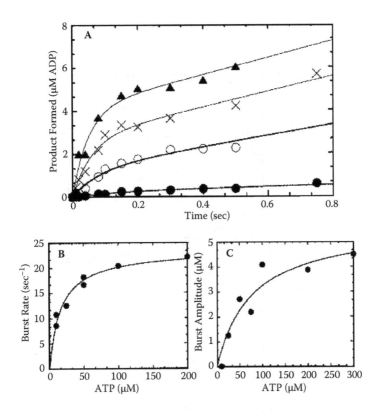

FIGURE 3.1 Experimental measurements of the temporal evolution of ADP in enzymatic hydrolysis of ATP by kinesin-related Ncd motor proteins at different initial concentrations of ATP. (A) The increase in the amount of ADP as a function of time. The concentrations are (from top to bottom) 100 μM, 50 μM, 25 μM, and 10 μM. (B) Burst rates as a function of initial ATP concentrations. (C) Burst amplitudes as a function of initial ATP concentrations. The figure is adapted with permission from Foster and Gilbert 2000 [56]. Copyright 2000 American Chemical Society.

of the end group depends on the local environment, so that the amplitude of the signal varied with the distance between helicase and the end group. Experimental results are presented in Figs. 3.2a and 3.2b for DNA segments of different nucleotide length. One can see that the fluorescent signal increased faster for shorter DNA segments, and the peak was corresponding to the motor protein reaching the end of the DNA chain. The subsequent decrease in the fluorescent signal for longer times was associated with dissociation of the helicase from the DNA molecule. From these experiments the rate of fluorescence changes was connected with specific chemical transitions associated with functioning of PcrA motor proteins including protein binding and unbinding from DNA, the translocation rate, the hydrolysis rate, and rates of hydrolysis products release (Dillingham et al. 2002) [43].

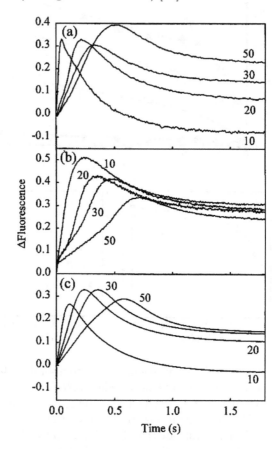

FIGURE 3.2 The change in fluorescence as a function of time for translocation of PcrA helicase motor proteins along DNA segments of different length. The numbers correspond to the length of oligonucleotides. (a) Preformed helicase–DNA complexes were mixed with ATP. (b) Helicase molecules were mixed with DNA oligonucleotides and with ATP. (c) Computer simulations of kinetic model for translocation. The figure is adapted with permission from Dillingham et al. 2002 [43]. Copyright 2002 American Chemical Society.

The stopped-flow method is a very convenient kinetic method of monitoring biochemical processes in motor proteins because it provides a continuous record of the process. A large number of experiments can be performed very quickly. However, there are also many limitations of this method. There is a time period after mixing all components and before the data are collected, which can be on the order of ~1 ms. Hence, the method cannot capture very fast chemical processes. In addition, fluorescently labeled molecules that are required might change the kinetic properties of motor proteins because of the fluorescent groups that must be attached to them. However, the biggest problem of the method is the interpretation of results. One has to assume some reaction scheme and fit the data, and it is not always successful. One can see this from Fig. 3.2c where results of computer simulations of a specific kinetic model to describe the translocation of PcrA helicase are presented. The comparison with experimental data suggests that this kinetic model provides only a fairly poor qualitative agreement.

In general, there is one serious flaw of all bulk chemical-kinetic methods. They measure average properties of a large number of motor protein molecules, while some of them might be more active and some of them are less active. This dynamic heterogeneity complicates the determination of the mechanisms of molecular motors at the single-molecule level. However, these measurements are very important as a tool that quantifies in what specific biochemical transitions motor proteins participate.

3.3   STRUCTURAL STUDIES

To determine microscopic mechanisms of motor proteins, one needs to know the positions of all atoms in these molecules. This assists in identification of the most relevant inter-atomic interactions that drive chemical and mechanical transitions in biological motors. This information is provided by structural methods (Howard 2001, Rice et al. 1999, Sweeney and Houdusse 2010, Roberts et al. 2013, Vale 2003, Marx et al. 2005, Marx et al. 2009, Kozielski et al. 1997, Liu et al. 2006, Engel et al. 2013, Singleton et al. 2007) [68, 132, 161, 133, 172, 107, 106, 88, 94, 49, 148]. There are two main experimental approaches, X-ray crystallography and cryomicroscopy, that are currently widely used in analyzing structures of various motor protein molecules.

X-ray crystallography is one of the most powerful and well-established experimental tools for structure determination (Rupp 2009) [137]. It was developed a century ago and it is based on a diffraction of X-ray radiation by electrons in the crystal material. It was shown in 1914 by British physicists W.H. Bragg and his son W.L. Bragg that because crystals are composed of periodic arrays of identical atoms, the scattering of X-rays could be viewed as a reflection from periodic planes of atoms within a crystal. Electrons in each atom change the direction of incoming X-rays, and these scattered waves produce specific diffraction patterns. It was suggested then that the analysis of these diffraction patterns can be utilized for determining positions of atoms in crystals. The importance of this method was immediately realized and both father and son Braggs received the Nobel Prize in Physics in 1915. It had a strong impact in advancing our knowledge of biological systems. The most famous example is the discovery of the DNA double-helix structure by Watson and Crick after analyzing X-ray diffraction data on crystals of Na salts of DNA. The interesting story here is that actual high-quality X-ray diffraction photographs of DNA were obtained first by Maurice Wilkins (a New Zealand–

born English physicist) who shared with Watson and Crick in 1962 a Nobel Prize for Physiology and Medicine for discovery of the molecular structure of nucleic acids.

X-ray crystallography turned out to be also important for investigations of motor proteins (Howard 2001, Rice et al. 1999, Sweeney and Houdusse 2010, Roberts et al. 2013, Vale 2003, Marx et al. 2005, Marx et al. 2009, Kozielski et al. 1997, Liu et al. 2006, Engel et al. 2013, Singleton et al. 2007) [68, 132, 161, 133, 172, 107, 106, 88, 94, 49, 148]. The crystal structure of the dimeric conventional kinesin obtained in 1997 is presented in Fig. 3.3 (Kozielski et al. 1997) [88]. The high quality of this structure allowed researchers to understand many features of kinesin behavior (Marx et al. 2009) [106]. Another example of a highly informative crystal structure of motor proteins is given in Fig. 2.9 where the structure of RNA polymerase is shown.

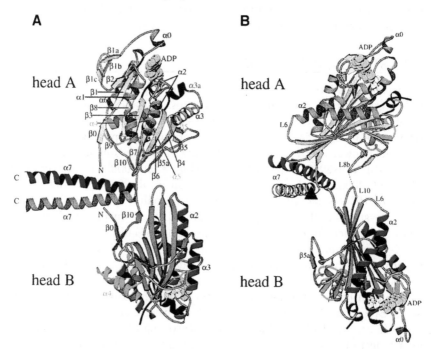

FIGURE 3.3 Structure of dimeric kinesin molecules obtained by X-ray crystallography method. Motor domains, neck linker, and part of the neck coiled-coil domains are shown. Two molecular views (A and B) differ by rotation around 65 degrees with respect to each. The figure is adapted with permission from Kozielski et. al. 1997 [88].

The method of X-ray crystallography is currently the most precise technique of obtaining structural information. It provides images of various biochemical states of molecular motors with atomic-scale resolutions. However, there are many issues associated with this method. First of all, one has to obtain protein crystals, but for various reasons, less than 30% of protein molecules can be crystallized. Even for situations when protein crystals exist it is not clear how realistic are molecular structures obtained in X-ray crystallography. This is because in many cases the experimental conditions differ significantly from cellular conditions (Kolomeisky 2013) [82]. For example, the most stable molecular structure at 0 °C and below (where crystals are observed) might not correctly represent dominating protein conformations at 37 °C (typical cellular conditions). In addition, X-ray crystallography provides only static information (atomic positions are frozen), while for understanding the mechanisms of biological molecular motors, a dynamic input is highly desirable.

A related structural method is a cryo-electron microscopy when the biological samples are investigated at very low temperatures (typically, these cryogenic conditions are created by liquid nitrogen) with transmission electron microscopes (Frank 2006, Milne et al. 2013) [57, 113]. In these experiments, passing electron beams are scattered differently by atoms in the sample, and electronic density maps are produced. From these data, the atomic structures are obtained via mathematically complex reconstruction procedures (Milne et al. 2013) [113], which is also true for X-ray crystallography. The advantage of cryomicroscopy over X-ray crystallography is that samples are prepared at natural physiological conditions.

However, the resolution is lower, and to get reasonable information from these measurements they need to be combined with data from X-ray crystallography and other spectroscopic techniques. In addition, the measurements are made at very low temperatures where protein molecular structures might strongly deviate from structures observed at typical cellular conditions. To show the capabilities of this method for motor proteins, the obtained structure of the bacterial flagellar motor is shown in Fig. 3.4 (Suzuki et al. 2004) [158]. One should notice that generally in cryomicroscopy one cannot obtain images without significant efforts in image reconstruction, which can frequently lead to artefacts and errors (Milne et al. 2013) [113]. Furthermore, this method gives only static properties of motor proteins.

Recently another powerful method of *nuclear magnetic resonance* (NMR) was introduced for structural studies in motor protein systems (Tzeng et al. 2012) [168]. NMR is based on identification of the local chemical environment for specific atoms due to interactions of their nuclear spins with applied magnetic fields. However, the method is still very complicated and expensive, which limits its application for biological molecular motors.

3.4 SINGLE-MOLECULE FORCE SPECTROSCOPY

We want to understand the microscopic mechanisms of motor proteins, but this can only be accomplished if properties of single molecules can be reliably measured. This opportunity was not available to researchers until 1990s

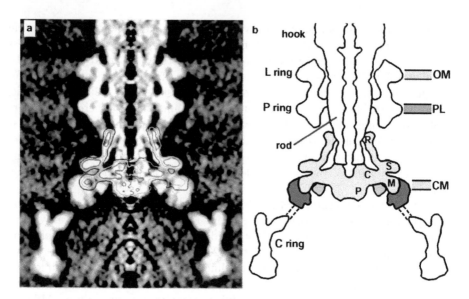

FIGURE 3.4   A) Superimposed contoured density maps of the rotor part of bacterial flagellar motor from cryoEM images of separate regions. B) A schematic drawing of the main part of the rotary motor protein. The figure is adapted with permission from Suzuki et. al. 2004 [158].

when the development of new single-molecule experimental methods and their applications to molecular motors started (Howard 2001, Kolomeisky and Fisher 2007, Chowdhury 2013, Veigel and Schmidt 2011, Greenleaf et al. 2007, Kolomeisky 2013, Dulin et al. 2013) [68, 84, 30, 175, 63, 82, 46]. Currently, there are many powerful techniques that might be used to interrogate motor protein dynamics, including optical-trap spectrometry, magnetic tweezers spectroscopy, Förster resonance energy transfer (FRET), single-molecule atomic-force microscopy (AFM), fluorescent labeling, super-resolution spectroscopy, and many other methods (Berg 2004, Greenleaf et al. 2007, Veigel and Schmidt 2011, Neuman and Nagy 2008, Dulin et al. 2013) [19, 63, 175, 118, 46]. These experimental approaches provide a powerful tool for investigating biological molecular motors with very high spatial and temporal resolutions. They have also given us the largest amount of information concerning the microscopic mechanisms of motor proteins. Let us discuss some of these single-molecule methods and what properties of molecular motors they have measured. We will concentrate on single-molecule force spectroscopy techniques, and their capabilities are summarized and compared in Table 3.1. The main feature of these methods is a precise measurement of forces produced or experienced by biological molecular motors.

TABLE 3.1   Comparing Single-Molecule Force Spectroscopy Methods

	Optical Traps	Magnetic Tweezers	AFM
Spatial Resolution	0.1–1 nm	5–10 nm	0.5–1 nm
Time Resolution	0.1 ms	1–10 ms	1 ms
Force Range	0.1–100 pN	0.01–100 pN	$10–10^4$ pN
Length Scales	$0.1–10^4$ nm	$10–10^4$ nm	$1–10^4$ nm
Probe Size	0.2–1 μ m	0.5–5 μ m	100–250 μ m
Advantages	High resolution 3D control	Constant force Rotations Specific	Imaging Bond breaking
Limitations	Photodamage Sample heating Nonspecific	No manipulation Bulky handles	Nonspecific Large forces

3.4.1   Optical-Trap Spectroscopy

The most powerful and advanced single-molecule force spectroscopy technique is known as *optical-trap* or *optical-tweezers spectroscopy* (Greenleaf et al. 2007, Veigel and Schmidt 2011, Neuman and Nagy 2008) [63, 175, 118]. It has been widely utilized in measuring dynamic properties of various single motor protein molecules (Svoboda et al. 1993, Svoboda and Block 1994, Finer et al. 1994, Visscher et al. 1999, Schnitzer et al. 2000, Mehta et al. 1999, Nishiyama et al. 2002, Uemura et al. 2004, Carter and Cross 2005, Toba et al. 2006) [160, 159, 53, 177, 142, 110, 99, 169, 27, 165]. The method is based on very precise monitoring of displacements of a bead that is chemically attached to a single motor protein molecule (Howard 2001, Veigel and Schmidt 2011, Greenleaf et al. 2007) [68, 175, 63]. The bead is controlled by an external non-uniform laser field which pushes it to the focus of the laser beam, as shown in Figs. 1.3 and 3.5. This trapping is the most important ingredient of the method.

The origin of this force can be understood by analyzing Fig. 3.5. The light coming into the spherical bead can be viewed as a flux of tiny particles that are called *photons*. The bead changes the direction of light photons because of the different refraction index of the material of the bead: see Fig. 3.5. The refraction (change of direction) is due to different velocities of the light in the bead and outside. This process is associated then with a change in the total momentum of the system, and this difference in momentum leads to the appearance of an effective force — recall Newton's Second Law. There are more photons from the region of the laser field with higher intensity so they produce larger force (Fig. 3.5). As a result, there is an optical force that pushes the bead in the direction of the stronger field, which corresponds to the focus region in optical-trap experiments. The effective potential created by the non-uniform laser field on the bead is very close to a harmonic potential. In other words, the optical force, like a spring, depends linearly on the distance from the focus. This allows a very precise calibration of force measurements. One can also independently monitor the motion of the bead with very high precision. In these experiments only the motion of the bead could be observed. The diameters of beads range from several hundred nanometers to a micron. The molecular motors are much smaller (~ 1–10 nm) and they cannot be seen. But the motor protein molecules are tightly bound to the bead, so it is assumed that they strongly follow the bead translocations. This allows researchers to obtain a lot of information on dynamic properties of biological molecular motors.

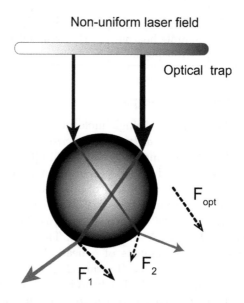

Non-uniform laser field

Optical trap

F_{opt}

F_1

F_2

FIGURE 3.5   The appearance of an optical force in the optical-trap experiments. Photons from the higher-intensity region of the field produce a larger force (F_1) due to the momentum change, while the weaker-intensity region produces a weaker force (F_2). The resulting optical force F_{opt} is a vectorial sum of all forces from all photons coming through the spherical bead. It has a horizontal component in the direction of the higher-intensity region.

To illustrate better the operation of the optical-trap systems, we present an experimental setup and typical particle trajectories in Fig. 3.6a. The original optical tweezers method was significantly advanced when a force clamp was added (Finer et al. 1994) [53]. By maintaining a constant distance between the focus of the laser field and the bead at all times (via electronic feedback system), researchers were able to monitor dynamics of motor proteins at constant external forces. As one can see from Fig. 3.6b, the difference in the distances between the optical trap and the bead never exceeded more than 10 nm, which corresponds to measuring forces with a very impressive precision of less than 0.5 pN. The optical trap technique was further improved by adding additional optical traps and by including measurements of forces in all directions (so-called vectorial loads) (Greenleaf et al. 2007, Veigel and Schmidt 2011) [63, 175]. It has been suggested that the most advanced versions of the optical-trap methods could reach a spatial resolution close to 0.1 nm (typical size of chemical bonds), and that biochemical transitions lasting not more than ~ 100 μs could also be successfully resolved (Greenleaf et al. 2007, Veigel and Schmidt 2011) [63, 175]. In addition, the method could provide a means of directly exerting forces on single molecules in the range from 0.1 pN up to 100 pN. But the strongest advantage of using optical-trap spectroscopy is the fact that it can be easily coupled with a variety of other methods such as FRET and other fluorescence labeling approaches (Greenleaf et al. 2007, Veigel and Schmidt 2011) [63, 175].

Currently, the optical trap approach is most successful and the most popular technique in elucidating dynamic properties of motor proteins. However, the method has several drawbacks and limitations that researchers should know about. It is very difficult to apply optical traps spectroscopy for studying processes in live cells, although there are several examples where it was accomplished (Greenleaf et al. 2007, Veigel and Schmidt 2011, Neuman and Nagy 2008) [63, 175, 118]. The most advanced and precise optical tweezers methods involve a very complex experimental geometry that might not be easily created for studying complex cellular processes. In addition, in these experiments we can only see the motion of optical beads, and assume that this provides a correct dynamic description of the attached motor proteins. In biological cells the presence of other molecules and cellular objects (cytoskeleton, membranes, vesicles) might change the overall dynamics. The bead might collide with other molecules or even bind to them for some extended period of time, which will definitely affect the interpretation of experimental data. The optical trap system is not very selective. It will trap any other dielectric particle, distorting measurements. For this reason the most precise experiments have been performed at very diluted solutions. Another problem of optical tweezers is a local heating due to the high intensity of the laser field. Changes in the temperature of the solution even for a few degrees can lead to very large modifications of enzymatic activities supported by motor proteins.

3.4.2 *Magnetic Tweezers Spectroscopy*

Magnetic tweezers spectroscopy is another method closely related to the optical-trap microscopy that was successfully utilized for investigating biological molecular motors (De Vlaminck and Dekker 2012, Greenleaf et al. 2007, Veigel and Schmidt 2011, Neuman and Nagy 2008) [73, 63, 175, 118]. This is a relatively simple and easy-to-implement approach which is based on applying a magnetic field to paramagnetic beads that are coupled to motor protein molecules (De Vlaminck and Dekker 2012, Neuman and Nagy 2008) [73, 118]: see Fig. 3.7. In these experiments the investigated molecules (motor

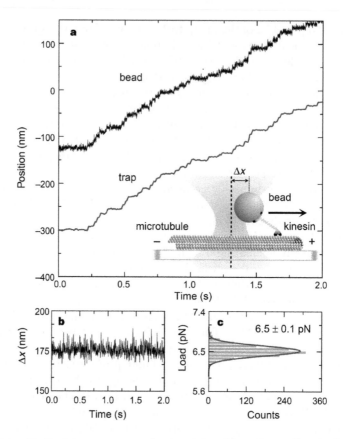

FIGURE 3.6   Optical trap measurements with a force clamp for single kinesin molecules. (a) A typical trajectory of the bead and of the focus of the laser field labeled as a trap at high ATP concentration. Inset shows a schematic picture of experimental setup. (b) Distance between the trap and the bead as a function of time during optical-trap measurements. (c) Force exerted by the optical trap calculated from the experiments. The figure is adapted with permission from Visscher et al. 1999 [177].

proteins or nucleic acids bound to motor proteins) are simultaneously chemically connected to the surface and to the magnetic particle. Large magnets positioned above the system generate the magnetic moment on the bead (see Fig. 3.7). The force experienced by the bead is proportional to the gradient of the magnetic field, and in most cases it is almost a constant for a large range of bead displacements. Thus experiments in magnetic tweezers systems are always done in force-clamp conditions, which is a great advantage of the method. Magnets producing the field can be rotated and it allows for the bead to exert torques on attached molecules. Using video microscopy the vertical position z of the bead, as well as the horizontal fluctuations parallel to the surface, $< x^2 >$, are determined (Neuman and Nagy 2008) [118]. Assuming that the surface-bound molecule exerts the elastic force on the bead in the vertical direction, $F_z = kz$, one can use the equipartition theorem that estimates this elastic energy at temperature T as equal to $\frac{1}{2}k_BT$ ($k_B = 1.3810^{-23}$ J/K is the *Boltzmann constant*),

$$\frac{1}{2}k\langle x^2 \rangle = \frac{1}{2}k_BT. \tag{3.4}$$

This leads to an expression for the axial force in magnetic tweezers experiments,

$$F_z = \frac{zk_BT}{\langle x^2 \rangle}. \tag{3.5}$$

The magnetic tweezers approach has several advantages over the optical-trap spectrometry (De Vlaminck and Dekker 2012, Greenleaf et al. 2007, Veigel and Schmidt 2011, Neuman and Nagy 2008) [73, 63, 175, 118]. The experimental setup does not lead to undesired overheating and photodamage. In addition, the method is very selective since only paramagnetic beads can be affected by the magnetic field, providing a convenient way of doing measurements in complex heterogeneous systems. This technique can be parallelized, allowing measurements of large number of molecules while still remaining sensitive to the complexity of the system. This is very convenient for investigating rare events which are found in many cellular processes. It can also be coupled with other single-molecule approaches, including optical traps and fluorescence labeling methods. But the biggest advantage of magnetic tweezers is the ability of exerting rotations and applying large torques (up to ~ 1000 pN nm^{-1}) and twists to biological molecules. It allowed researchers to investigate with a high resolution the functioning of multiple nucleic acid motor proteins, such as topoisomerases, gyrases, and others, for which rotational degrees of freedom are critically important. For example, magnetic tweezers have been used to explore the details of how topoisomerase motor proteins help to relax supercoiled DNA molecules by removing the topological defects; see Fig. 3.7.

However, there are also many limitations and drawbacks in magnetic tweezers spectroscopy (De Vlaminck and Dekker 2012, Greenleaf et al. 2007, Veigel and Schmidt 2011, Neuman and Nagy 2008) [73, 63, 175, 118]. The bead monitoring system generally has a lower temporal and spatial resolution than the optical-trap method. Dynamic properties of motor proteins are obtained indirectly by measuring the molecular extensions. For example, observing the change in the supercoiled DNA length will not provide information on the position of the topoisomerase and on how they remove the topological defects (Fig. 3.7). In addition, the precise measurements of the force in these experiments is based on employing the equilibrium concept of equipartition. But the investigated biological systems are almost always far away from equilibrium, and the application of equipartition theorem might not be reliable.

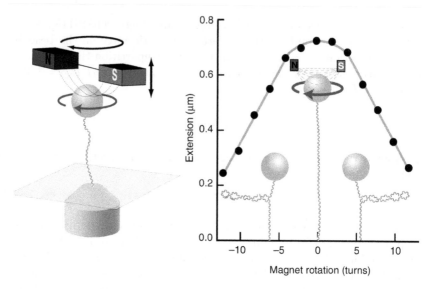

FIGURE 3.7   Left: A schematic view of the basic setup for magnetic tweezers experiments. The paramagnetic bead is connected to the surface by the biological molecule (nucleic acids with motors or motor proteins). Permanent magnets above the experimental chamber produce a force on the bead in the vertical direction. A rotation of magnets can create torques. The video microscopy system below the experimental chamber tracks the real-time position of the bead. Right: Experimental measurements for coiling and unwinding of DNA molecules. The removal of twist in DNA is accomplished by topoisomerase motor proteins. The action of these motor proteins can be seen by monitoring the extension from the bead to the surface. The figure is adapted with permission from Neuman and Nagy 2008 [118].

3.4.3   *Atomic-Force Microscopy*

A much simpler physical concept is utilized in another very useful and widely applied single-molecule method known as *atomic-force microscopy* (AFM) (Greenleaf et al. 2007, Veigel and Schmidt 2011, Neuman and Nagy 2008) [63, 175, 118]. A basic setup consists of a cantilever with a sharp tip to which a biomolecule is attached (see Fig. 3.8). The motion of the cantilever is recorded by using a deflection of a laser beam, and the vertical motion of the probe is controlled by a piezoelectric mechanical actuator. The cantilever can be viewed as a linear spring, and from its bending the elastic force can be estimated; see Fig. 3.8. In single-molecule AFM experiments the stiffness of the utilized cantilever typically varies from 10 to 10^5 pN/nm. The results of AFM measurements are high-resolution force-versus-extension curves of single molecules (Greenleaf et al. 2007, Veigel and Schmidt 2011, Neuman and

Nagy 2008, Kodera et al. 2010) [63, 175, 118, 119]. Information on molecular mechanisms is derived by analyzing these experimental data.

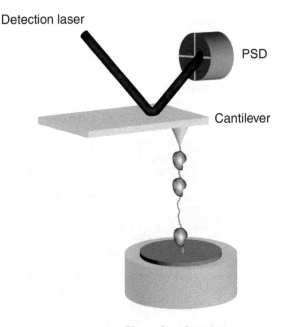

Detection laser

PSD

Cantilever

Piezoelectric scanner

FIGURE 3.8   A schematic view of atomic force microscopy experiments. A molecule is chemically attached to the cantilever with a sharp tip. Its motion is monitored by a position-sensitive detector (PSD) which measures the deflection of the laser beam. The piezoelectric stage is moved vertically to change the separation between the cantilever and the molecule. The figure is adapted with permission from Neuman and Nagy 2008 [118].

In studies of biological molecular motors, this experimental approach has been used for probing folding/unfolding dynamics of several proteins (Greenleaf et al. 2007, Veigel and Schmidt 2011, Neuman and Nagy 2008) [63, 175, 118]. In addition, it was successful in the imaging of kinesin and myosin V motors during their motion on cytoskeleton filaments as shown in Fig. 3.9 (Veigel and Schmidt 2011, Kodera et al. 2010) [175, 119]. One could even see the motion of individual protein domains. This provided important clues for deciphering mechanisms of motor proteins motility. It showed that AFM spectroscopy is a valuable tool in probing dynamic properties and interactions with other biological objects for biological molecular motors, and it can be coupled with other single-molecule methods to make it even more useful (Greenleaf et al. 2007, Veigel and Schmidt 2011, Neuman and Nagy 2008) [63, 175, 118].

Nevertheless, AFM methods also have their own drawbacks and limitations. Due to a relatively high stiffness of the cantilever, only large forces (between 10 pN and 10^4 pN) can be exerted. For most motor proteins weaker forces are usually observed. In addition, the selectivity is quite low in AFM pulling experiments. Other molecules present in the system could bind to the cantilever affecting its motion, and this cannot be easily discriminated. The size of the tip is quite large (hundreds of microns), and this leads to large thermal fluctuations as well as stronger effects from local changes in viscosity. As a result, the resolution of AFM methods is frequently low, especially in comparison with optical-trap and magnetic tweezers techniques.

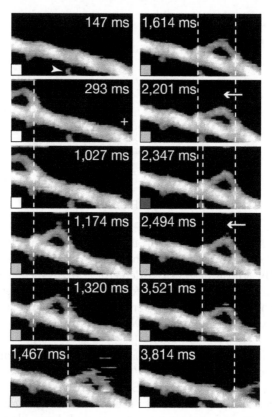

FIGURE 3.9 AFM images of walking along actin filament myosin V motor protein molecule at different times. One can clearly see two motor domains of bound to the cytoskeleton filament. The figure is adapted with permission from Kodera et al. 2010 [119].

It is interesting to compare different single-molecule force spectroscopy methods, and their major properties, as already discussed above, are presented in Table 3.1. From this analysis one can conclude that the application of single-molecule force spectroscopy methods is crucial for obtaining a comprehensive picture of motor proteins activities in cellular systems. However, one should be critical in evaluating experimental observations, and a combination of different methods should be used in deducing possible mechanisms of biological molecular motors.

3.5 FLUORESCENT LABELING AND SUPER-RESOLUTION TECHNIQUES

To determine mechanisms and dynamics of molecular motors, not only the information on forces and torques that they produce is required, but one should also know the spatial positions of the various protein domains and groups at different times. This kind of information is supplied by light microscopy techniques that utilize fluorescent labels (Greenleaf et al. 2007, Veigel and Schmidt 2011, Yildiz et. al. 2003) [63, 175, 184]. In these experiments small chemical molecules that fluoresce at typical conditions (called *fluorescent dyes*) are attached to specific positions on motor protein molecules. This allows one to localize and track single motors with a high resolution by looking at these fluorescent labels in an optical microscope.

To illustrate the single-molecule fluorescent labeling method, let us consider experiments in which single fluorophores were bound to a myosin V motor protein traveling on actin cytoskeleton filaments (Yildiz et al. 2003) [184]. The fluorescent dye was attached to the motor domain on the protein, while actin filaments were immobilized on a surface to improve the resolution. Fluorescent images at different times were collected and analyzed as shown in Fig. 3.10. Associating the brightest part of the fluorescent spot with a position of the dye attached to the motor domain, dynamics of myosin V stepping was directly visualized and quantified. These experiments show that fluorescent labeling for investigating biological molecular motors is very powerful.

However, there are several known limitations of this approach (Greenleaf et al. 2007, Veigel and Schmidt 2011) [63, 175]. The temporal resolution is not very high ($\sim 100~\mu s$) so that fast conformational changes in motor proteins cannot be captured. Another problem is the fact that the label will eventually stop fluorescing (the process is known as a *photobleaching*), and this limits the experimental time. It is important also to check that attaching the dye group does not significantly change the properties of investigated motor proteins. In addition, only very diluted systems can be analyzed because binding of other molecules can frequently quench the fluorescence of label groups. But this might not be a realistic description of cellular conditions under which motor proteins function. Furthermore, a very large number of photons must be collected to obtain high spatial resolutions.

There is one very serious problem in application of fluorescent methods for understanding dynamics of single molecular motors. It is related to a fundamental limit in the spatial resolution that can be achieved in these experiments (Toomre and Bewersdorf 2010, Schermelleh et al. 2010, Saka and Rizzoli 2012)

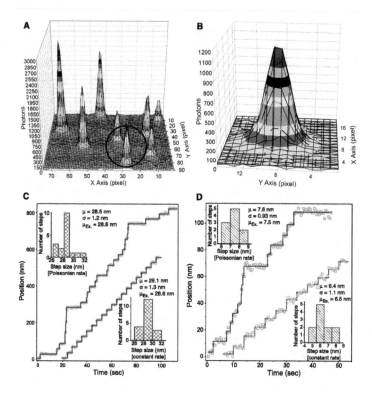

FIGURE 3.10   (A) Photon distribution functions for fluorescent-labeled myosin V motors. (B) Fitting of the photon distribution functions to enable the localization of the peak. (C) and (D) Stepping traces of fluorescent dyes connected to the myosin V motor protein. The figure is adapted with permission from Yildiz et al. 2003 [184].

[166, 141, 139]. Since the light is utilized to interrogate biological systems, the size of the object to be observed cannot be much smaller than the wavelength λ of the light. This is known as a *diffraction limit*. In simple terms, the physical origin of the diffraction barrier is the fact that the image of the point source of light is a combination of different incoming waves. The waves that differ by integer number of wavelengths ($n\lambda$ with $n = 1, 2, \ldots$) will combine and they will be seen, but waves that differ by half wavelength ($n\lambda/2$ with $n = 1, 2, \ldots$) will cancel each other. As a result, the image of the point source of light has a size proportional to the wavelength. For currently used experimental methods it turns out that this limit is above ~ 200 nm, which is too large for obtaining detailed information on biological molecular motors. Fortunately, several ways to resolve this problem were presented recently, leading to a development of new experimental methods known as super-resolution spectroscopy (Toomre and Bewersdorf 2010, Schermelleh et al. 2010, Saka and

TABLE 3.2   Comparison of Super-Resolution Microscopy Methods

	SIM	STED	PALM/STORM
Spatial Resolution	50–100 nm	10–100 nm	20–50 nm
Time Resolution	1–1000 ms	1–1000 ms	1–100 s
Photobleaching	Moderate	High	High
Data Processing	Required	Not required	Required
Advantages	Simple setup	High resolution No data processing	High resolution Simple setup
Limitations	Low resolution Data processing	Fluorophores	Fluorophores Data processing

Rizzoli 2012) [166, 141, 139]. The importance of the super-resolution methods for investigating complex chemical and biological systems was recognized in the 2014 Nobel Prize in Chemistry, awarded to the founders of this approach W.E. Moerner, S. Hell, and E. Betzig.

There are three main super-resolution methods that are widely employed in studies of various biological systems (Toomre and Bewersdorf 2010, Schermelleh et al. 2010, Saka and Rizzoli 2012, Meyer et al. 2008) [166, 141, 139, 111]. They include: (1) *structural illumination microscopy* (SIM); (2) *stimulated emission depletion* (STED); and a set of two related techniques known as (3) *photoactivated localization microscopy* (PALM) and *stochastic optical reconstruction microscopy* (STORM). The properties of different approaches are compared in Table 3.2. The most serious limitations for all methods are their large complexity and extremely high cost of experiments.

The idea of the super-resolution method SIM is the following (Toomre and Bewersdorf 2010, Schermelleh et al. 2010, Saka and Rizzoli 2012) [166, 141, 139]. The biological sample is imaged together with a pattern of fine stripes, which is varied in space and time. The distances between stripes are usually smaller than the diffraction limit. Then combining several images followed by a mathematical reconstruction that analyzes the signal variations allows researchers to obtain a high-resolution view of the investigated biological object. However, the spatial resolution improvement is limited, and the best SIM techniques cannot visualize objects that are smaller than ~ 50 nm. In addition, the temporal resolution is quite low.

STED microscopy is a more popular super-resolution method that uses two overlapping laser beams (Toomre and Bewersdorf 2010, Schermelleh et al. 2010, Saka and Rizzoli 2012, Meyer et al. 2008) [166, 141, 139, 111]. One of them excites the fluorophores attached to the biological object, while another one is a longer-wavelength light that has a donut shape form with tiny hole (smaller than the diffraction limit) in the middle. The role of the second laser is to quench the fluorescence of the sample everywhere except at the central hole area. Thus STED deactivates the fluorophore activity at the periphery of the investigated object, leading to a significantly larger spatial resolution

(10–30 nm). The results of the application of this technique to a biological system of neurofilaments are shown in Fig. 3.11.

Despite the success of this method in many biological systems, there are several limitations and drawbacks. Unfortunately, there is a very small choice of fluorophore groups that might be utilized in STED. In addition, it is quite difficult to set up experiments with multiple colors, i.e., to utilize fluorophores with different wavelengths.

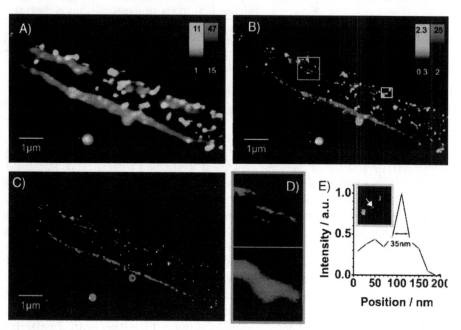

FIGURE 3.11   (A) Image obtained by classical confocal microscopy. (B) Image obtained by STED microscopy. (C) Improved analysis of STED image. (D) The smaller area images from confocal and STED microscopy. One can see that the STED image reveals a strand structure that is not seen in the confocal picture. (E) Improved spatial resolution. The figure is adapted with permission from Meyer et al. 2008 [111].

A very different approach is employed in PALM/STORM super-resolution methods (Toomre and Bewersdorf 2010, Schermelleh et al. 2010, Saka and Rizzoli 2012) [166, 141, 139]. Here, an idea similar to analysis of photon distribution functions in single fluorescent molecule experiments (Yildiz et al. 2003) [184], as described above, is applied again. The brightest center of the image can be resolved with a very high resolution if a significantly large number of photons is collected. In addition, fluorescent labels are randomly switched on and off, and the mathematical analysis of images obtained at different times leads to higher spatial resolution ($\sim$ 20–30 nm). These methods have been successfully used for tracking various motor proteins in *in vitro* systems as well as in live cells (Veigel and Schmidt 2011) [175]. Nevertheless, the main problems of PALM/STORM methods again include a very limited set of fluorophores that can be used and low temporal resolutions. Despite these issues, it is widely expected that all super-resolution methods will be exploited in the future as a powerful tool for uncovering properties of motor proteins.

3.6   MAJOR EXPERIMENTAL OBSERVATIONS

A large volume of information on structural, biochemical, and dynamic properties of biological molecular motors have been obtained using a variety of experimental methods. We already discussed the advantages and limitations of several techniques. Here we present some experimental findings for specific motor protein systems.

It was found that conventional kinesins are processive motor proteins that travel along microtubules in the plus direction of the filament with speeds reaching up to 1 μm/s (Svoboda et al. 1993, Svoboda and Block 1994, Visscher et al. 1999, Schnitzer et al. 2000, Carter and Cross 2005, Veigel and Schmidt 2011) [160, 159, 177, 142, 27, 175]. They usually make around $\sim$ 100 steps before they detach, and the length of each step is equal to $d = 8.2$ nm. It was shown that kinesins have a tight mechanochemical coupling, i.e., one molecule of ATP is consumed to make each mechanical step. During their motion, kinesins might produce forces up to 7–8 pN (Visscher et al. 1999, Schnitzer et al. 2000) [177, 142]. It corresponds to experimentally measured stall forces.

Experiments indicate that cytoplasmic dyneins are also processive motors that move along microtubules in the minus direction (Tobe et al. 2006, Gennerich and Vale 2009) [165, 59]. The step size of these motors varies: at most conditions $d = 8.2$ nm hoppings are seen (like in kinesins), while in some cases larger step sizes have also been observed (up to $\sim$ 32 nm). A significant fraction of backward steps have also been measured in dyneins. The stall forces needed to stop these motors are probably smaller than for kinesins, but these experimental observations remain controversial.

Another class of cytoskeleton motor proteins, myosins V and myosins VI, that move in opposite directions along actin filaments have also been well investigated by different methods (Finer et al. 1994, Mehta et al. 1999, Uemura et al. 2004, Yildiz et al. 2003, Spudich and Sivaramakrishnan 2010) [53, 110, 169, 184, 154]. Their steps sizes and stall forces were determined to be $d \simeq 36$ nm $F_S \simeq 1 - 2.5$ pN, respectively. Single-molecule experiments showed that the majority of cytoskeleton dimer motor proteins (kinesins, dyneins, and myosins V and VI) follow the so-called hand-over-hand mechanism in their motion along cytoskeleton filaments. In this mechanism the filament-bound protein domains alternate between leading and trailing positions, similar to the way people walk.

Experimental studies have determined a variety of dynamic properties for multiple motor protein systems (Veigel and Schmidt 2011, Visscher et al. 1999,

Schnitzer et al. 2000, Carter and Cross 2005, Uemura et al. 2004, Gennerich and Vale 2009) [175, 177, 142, 27, 169, 59]. In most cases the dependence of motor velocities on external loads (force-velocity curves), and ATP concentrations, spatial fluctuations have been measured quite well. One of the most important experimental findings is the observation that all studied chemical transitions in motor proteins are fully reversible (Kolomeisky 20013, Veigel and Schmidt 2011, Carter and Cross 2005) [82, 175, 27].

3.7 SUMMARY

In this chapter we discussed major experimental methods that have been utilized for investigating motor proteins and their properties. Our analysis focused on bulk chemical kinetics, structural methods, single-molecule force spectroscopy, fluorescent labeling methods, and super-resolution microscopy. We argued that chemical kinetic methods provide a quantitative analysis of relevant biochemical transitions in motor proteins, structural methods reveal valuable information on molecular geometry of motors, and single-molecule techniques allow us to measure dynamics and forces of individual motor protein molecules with high spatial and temporal resolutions. It was concluded that all these different techniques provide a comprehensive view of motor protein activities at different conditions.

The theoretical foundations, advantages, and limitations of each experimental approach have been critically discussed and compared in order to understand the reliability of obtained experimental observations on biological motors. Finally, the main experimental observations for various motor proteins systems were presented. The road is now open for developing theoretical concepts that are required for understanding mechanisms and dynamics of biological molecular motors.

CHAPTER 4

Fundamental Physical Concepts: Equilibrium Approaches

CONTENTS

4.1   INTRODUCTION

It is known that motor proteins convert a chemical energy into a mechanical motion (Lodish et al. 2007, Alberts et al. 2007, Howard 2001) [95, 4, 68]. In their work, biological molecular motors are involved in a large number of chemical reactions and in interactions with other biological molecules such as the cytoskeleton proteins, and with DNA, RNA, and other enzymes. The motors interact with different molecules and cellular structures via mechanical, electrostatic, hydrodynamic, and chemical forces. On top of this, it is always important to remember that motor proteins function in biological cells that are strongly non-equilibrium systems. These observations raise a lot of issues that need be analyzed and clarified if we want to understand mechanisms of motor proteins. Crucial questions are:

    1. How can we rationalize all the observations quantitatively?

    2. What does it mean to be in a system at equilibrium or out of equilibrium and how important is it for molecular motors?

    3. Why can chemical energy be transformed into mechanical work and what is the efficiency of this process?

    4. How does the participation in chemical processes influence the properties of motor proteins?

5. What is the role of external fields in changing molecular motor dynamics?

6. How can we best describe the dynamic properties of motor proteins?

To answer these questions we need to discuss several fundamental scientific concepts. Since motor proteins are engaged in heat transformations we need to talk about equilibrium thermodynamics. Statistical mechanics will help us to understand how to calculate macroscopic features of motor protein systems from their molecular properties and how to distinguish between equilibrium or non-equilibrium states of these systems. Enzymatics will provide a framework for explaining the catalytic properties of motor proteins. Motor protein dynamics will be assessed by employing theoretical knowledge of diffusion, chemical kinetics, free-energy landscapes, and random walks. These fundamental concepts will be discussed in this chapter and in the following chapters. Our search for a microscopic understanding of molecular motors can be compared with travel to a very remote village. To reach this place quickly and safely, one should use good maps and high-quality roads. The collection of these well-established fundamental concepts and ideas play the role of such maps and highways in our journey to uncover complex mechanisms of molecular motors.

4.2 BASIC EQUILIBRIUM THERMODYNAMICS

Thermodynamics is a science that describes transformations of heat and work. It is a macroscopic theory, which means that it explains only the properties of large numbers of molecules. Thermodynamics considers *systems* that are defined as macroscopic parts of the universe surrounded by a surface, which can be real or virtual. The central concept of thermodynamics is the idea of *energy*, which is a basic physical property for every system. Experiments can only measure changes in energy, but they are never able to estimate its absolute value. Every system can be described by a set of *thermodynamic variables* or *parameters* that includes temperature (T), pressure (P), volume (V), and many others. These are macroscopic properties that are averaged over large groups of molecules present in the system. These physical functions are employed for explaining transformations of heat and work.

Equilibrium thermodynamics is built on two postulates and two fundamental laws. These statements are the results of a large number of practical observations which have never been violated. We will take them as granted. The first postulate introduces the concept of a *thermodynamic equilibrium*. It argues that if there are no changes of external parameters at the surrounding surface, the system will transfer at large times into the equilibrium state. If we put, for example, kinesin motor proteins in the solution without adding ATP molecules and microtubules, the solution will not change for a very long time. So one can say that this system is in equilibrium. Strictly speaking, thermodynamics suggests that the equilibrium state for any system can be reached only after very long times, but for practical purposes in many instances we can assume that the system is in equilibrium after finite times if the above conditions of no changes in thermodynamic parameters are satisfied.

The second postulate introduces a *temperature* T defined as a measure of the degree of hotness for any system. If we bring two bodies with different temperatures together, the temperature of the warmer body falls while the colder body will warm up. This process continues until the temperatures of the two bodies become equal. Then it will no longer change. We can think of the temperature as a kind of "heat force." The equilibrium in this system is reached when these "forces" equalize.

Another fundamental concept in thermodynamics is that of *work*, W. There are many types of work, including mechanical, chemical, electric, and many others. It is important to be clear about the sign of the work. Here we use the convention that the work is negative ($W < 0$) if it is done by a system on its surroundings. The positive work, $W > 0$, corresponds to the work done by the surroundings on the system. Be warned that it is easy to be confused here! One might remember the following rule: in thermodynamics the positive work always leads to an increase the system's energy. When the volume of the system changes from V_A to V_B under the effect of an opposing pressure P we have,

$$W_{PV} = -\int_{V_A}^{V_B} PdV. \tag{4.1}$$

Here the pressure generally depends on the volume. For an expansion, $V_B > V_A$, the work is negative because the work is done by the system on its surroundings. If the volume is decreasing during this process, $V_B < V_A$, the work is positive by definition. It is convenient to illustrate the work graphically, as shown in Fig. 4.1. The area under the curve corresponds to the work done by the system. It also implies the important property of the work: it depends not only on initial and final states of the system but also on details of the process. Many possible curves between the initial and final states may apply, and the work (area under the curve) obviously will be different.

For motor proteins moving a cellular cargo against an external force $f(x)$ along the x axis, there is another type of mechanical work which we call the force-distance work,

$$W_{FD} = \int_{x_A}^{x_B} f(x)dx. \tag{4.2}$$

Generally, the force will be position-dependent. The work is positive if the external force resists the motor protein's motion because the energy of the system is increasing in this case.

We can also heat any system by adding the amount of heat Q. One can introduce then a function U, called the *internal energy*, whose change is given by

$$\Delta U = Q + W_{PV} + W_{FD} + W_{other} = Q + W, \tag{4.3}$$

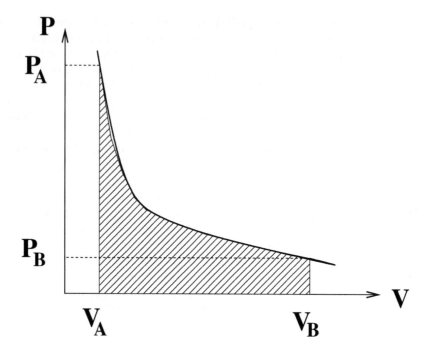

FIGURE 4.1 Graphical illustration of the pressure-volume work. The work is equal to the shaded area under the curve.

where W_{other} corresponds to all other types of work that the system can experience such as chemical, electric, magnetic, and surface work. U is defined as a system's *internal energy*. The First Law of Thermodynamics states that a change in U depends only on initial and final states of the system and it is independent of the process connecting them. It is also known as a *conservation-of-energy law*. One can see that for a process with the same initial and final states it is not possible to do work by the system without taking heat from outside. If during the process with different initial and final states the amount of heat exceeds the work done by the system, the internal energy of the system increases, $U = Q - (-W) > 0$. Similarly, for $Q < -W$ the internal energy will decrease.

Analyzing processes in thermodynamics, it is critical to make the following distinction. The heat Q and the work W depend on the process, whereas the change in the internal energy, ΔU, is fully specified by initial and final states of the system, no matter what path is taken by the system. The internal energy U is said to be a *state function*, while Q and W are not. For any process, a small incremental change in the work can be written as

$$dW = -PdV, \qquad (4.4)$$

and the full work for the process from the state A to the state B can be seen as a sum of such small increments,

$$W = \int_A^B dW. \tag{4.5}$$

The symbol d is called an *inexact derivative*. It simply means that the integral depends not only on initial and final states but also on the details of the process. This is in contrast with the exact differential dU that is used to describe the change in the internal energy,

$$\Delta U = U_B - U_A = \int_A^B dU. \tag{4.6}$$

Thermodynamics frequently employs the concept of *reversibility*. Here we assume that the process is reversible when the system proceeds through a sequence of equilibrium states (Widom 2002) [181]. The First Law of Thermodynamics can be conveniently written in the so-called differential form that describes the changes in thermodynamic parameters,

$$dU = dQ + dW, \tag{4.7}$$

which describes the incremental changes in these thermodynamic parameters. The dependence of Q and W on the pathway cancels out in the combination of these two thermodynamic quantities.

One can recognize that there are many processes in nature that occur spontaneously. One example was given above when we discussed what would happen if we bring together the hotter and the cooler objects. Another example is a diffusion of molecules from the region of higher concentration to the region of lower concentration. In all these cases, no work is done. This tendency to proceed spontaneously is associated with a very important function in thermodynamics which is called an *entropy*, S. More explicitly, the entropy is defined via

$$dQ_{rev} \leq T dS, \tag{4.8}$$

where the subscript "rev" indicates the heat in a reversible process. Note that while the heat depends on the details of the process, the entropy is a state function. One can see now that all terms for work can be viewed as products of generalized forces (P, f, ...) over generalized coordinates (V, x, ...), so we can extend this analogy to the entropy. It suggests that the entropy can be considered as a "heat coordinate."

There are many physical statements of the Second Law of Thermodynamics. One of them is the so-called *Clausius inequality*, which states that

$$dS \geq dQ/T, \tag{4.9}$$

for either reversible or irreversible processes. Thus, for isolated systems with no heat exchange ($dQ = 0$), the Second Law requires that

$$dS \geq 0. \tag{4.10}$$

This statement is also known as a *principle of entropy increase*. It suggests that all spontaneous processes move in the direction of entropy increase, and the maximal entropy is achieved at equilibrium where $dS = 0$.

Combining the First and Second Laws of Thermodynamics for a system where motor proteins move linearly against the external force $f(x)$, we can write

$$dU = TdS - PdV + fdx. \tag{4.11}$$

This equation describes all reversible mechanical and heat transformations. The state of the system is determined by the internal energy U which depends on thermodynamic parameters S, V_i and x. However, in chemistry, physics and biology it is inconvenient to use the entropy as a thermodynamic variable because it cannot be measured in experiments. It is much more practical to utilize chemical composition, temperature, pressure, and force since these parameters can be varied in experiments. To solve this problem, several other thermodynamic functions that specify the state of the system can be introduced. The most popular and convenient are *enthalpy, H*, *Helmholtz free energy, F*, and *Gibbs free energy, G*, which are defined as

$$H \equiv U + PV, \quad F \equiv U - TS, \quad G \equiv U - TS + PV. \tag{4.12}$$

It should be noted here that the development of major concepts and ideas in equilibrium thermodynamics is associated with a name of one of the most prominent American scientists J.W. Gibbs. He made many important contributions in different areas of physics, chemistry and mathematics. But the most interesting fact of his life is that he was the first recipient of a PhD degree in engineering in the United States! J.W. Gibbs obtained it in 1863 from Yale University (Fig. 4.2).

The combined expressions for the First and Second Laws of Thermodynamics for enthalpy, Helmholtz free energy and Gibbs free energy, can be written as

$$dH = TdS + VdP + fdx, \tag{4.13}$$

$$dF = -SdT - PdV + fdx, \tag{4.14}$$

$$dG = -SdT + VdP + fdx. \tag{4.15}$$

Especially convenient for analyzing the systems with chemical transformations is the Gibbs free energy, G. It can be argued that the spontaneous processes are taking place in the direction of lowering G, and the equilibrium state of any system is described by $dG = 0$, where the Gibbs free energy is minimal.

Now let us consider a system that has n moles of some chemical compound. If we add dn moles of the same compound to the system, the internal energy $U(S, V, x)$ will increase by the amount dU because the energy is proportional to the number of molecules in the system. We can then write

$$dU = \left(\frac{\partial U}{\partial S}\right)_{V,x,n} dS + \left(\frac{\partial U}{\partial V}\right)_{S,x,n} dV + \left(\frac{\partial U}{\partial x}\right)_{V,S,n} dx + \left(\frac{\partial U}{\partial n}\right)_{S,V,x} dn. \tag{4.16}$$

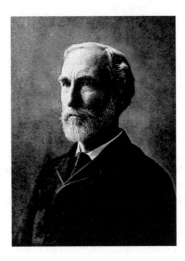

FIGURE 4.2   The famous American scientist Josiah Willard Gibbs (1839–1903) who developed and systematized the theoretical framework for equilibrium thermodynamics and statistical mechanics.

Comparing this expression with Eq. (4.11) the conclusion is that

$$T = \left(\frac{\partial U}{\partial S}\right)_{V,x,n}, \quad P = -\left(\frac{\partial U}{\partial V}\right)_{S,x,n}, \quad f = \left(\frac{\partial U}{\partial x}\right)_{V,S,n}. \qquad (4.17)$$

It suggests that derivatives of the internal energy U have a physical meaning of generalized forces for corresponding thermodynamic variables. It also allows us to define an important new function μ that is called a *chemical potential*,

$$\mu \equiv \left(\frac{\partial U}{\partial n}\right)_{S,V,x}. \qquad (4.18)$$

It has a meaning of a "chemical force" that drives changes in the composition of the system due to phase transitions or chemical reactions. The work to transfer n_i moles of the compound i to the system is equal to $dW_i = \mu_i dn_i$. For a process in a multi-component system (e.g., where chemical reactions are taking place) it can be also written as

$$dW_{chem} = \sum_i \mu_i dn_i. \qquad (4.19)$$

The chemical potential cannot be easily measured, but it can be calculated from other thermodynamic variables using the *Gibbs equation*. This equation is obtained by combining expressions for the First and Second Laws of Thermodynamics and accounting for the chemical work; specifically, one has

$$dG = -SdT + VdP + fdx + \sum_i \mu_i dn_i. \qquad (4.20)$$

This leads to another expression for the chemical potential in terms of the Gibbs free energy,

$$\mu_i = \left(\frac{\partial G}{\partial n_i} \right)_{T,P,x}. \tag{4.21}$$

One could show that the Gibbs free energy is given by

$$G = \sum_i \mu_i n_i. \tag{4.22}$$

Thus the Gibbs free energy is a sum of chemical potentials for all components of the system. So considering the system with only one type of molecule leads to an alternative definition of the chemical potential: it is just a Gibbs free energy per one mole, $\mu = G/n$. The majority of processes in chemistry and biology take place in solutions where it can be shown that for diluted solutions one can approximate the chemical potential of the component i in the following form,

$$\mu_i \simeq \mu_i^{(0)} + RT \ln c_i, \tag{4.23}$$

where $R = 8.31$ J/K is a fundamental quantity known as a *gas constant*, and c_i is the concentration of molecules of type i in the solution. The term $\mu_i^{(0)}$, which depends only on T, corresponds to the chemical potential for unit concentration of the compound i (i.e., for $c_i = 1$). Note, however, that for more concentrated solutions one should use activities rather than concentrations because of expected strong deviations from simple ideal behavior described here (Atkins and de Paula, 2009) [10].

Equilibrium thermodynamics provides a fundamental theoretical framework for understanding chemical reactions. To illustrate this, let us consider a system that can be described by just one chemical reaction. This is obviously a simplification since complex chemical and biological processes, including motor proteins, involve a large number of chemical reactions. In our simplified case, for the chemical reaction we can write the following scheme, which is also known as a *stoichiometric expression*,

$$\nu_1 A_1 + \nu_2 A_2 + \ldots = \nu_1' A_1' + \nu_2' A_2' + \ldots \tag{4.24}$$

In this equation $A_1, A_2, \ldots$ describe chemical formulas for various substances that participate in this process as the reactants, while the chemical formulas for products are given by $A_1', A_2', \ldots$. The parameters ν_i and ν_i' are stoichiometric coefficients that give the number of molecules or moles of each compound that was consumed or formed in this reaction. They are needed to keep the material balance in this chemical reaction: the total number of atoms of each type on the left side of the chemical reaction equation must be equal to the total number of the same atoms on the right side.

One can notice that the number of molecules of different components of the system are not independent. Defining dn_i and dn_i' as small changes in the number of moles for substances A_i (reactants) and A_i' (products) due to the chemical reaction expressed in Eq. (4.24) we have

$$\frac{dn_1}{\nu_1} = \frac{dn_2}{\nu_2} = \ldots = -\frac{dn_1'}{\nu_1'} = -\frac{dn_2'}{\nu_2'} = \ldots. \tag{4.25}$$

As an example, let us view the process of formation of water molecules by burning the hydrogen molecules in oxygen,

$$2H_2 + O_2 = 2H_2O. \tag{4.26}$$

In this case we have

$$\frac{dn_{H_2}}{2} = dn_{O_2} = -\frac{dn_{H_2O}}{2}. \tag{4.27}$$

This expression has a simple interpretation: every two molecules of hydrogen react with one molecule of oxygen to create 2 molecules of water. Thus we define a new variable ξ that can describe the progress of this chemical reaction,

$$d\xi = \frac{dn_i}{\nu_i} = -\frac{dn_i'}{\nu_i'}, \tag{4.28}$$

where $0 \leq \xi \leq 1$. The $\xi = 0$ corresponds to the case when only reactants are present and no products, while $\xi = 1$ marks the situation when the reaction is fully complete with only product substances present in the system. The parameter ξ is called a *chemical variable*, and it is very convenient for analyzing chemical reactions. Instead of monitoring changes in concentrations of many chemical compounds, we have one variable that can fully describe the degree of completeness for any chemical reaction. The Gibbs equation for this system can be written as

$$dG = -SdT + VdP + fdx + d\xi \left(\sum_i (\mu_i \nu_i - \mu_i' \nu_i') \right). \tag{4.29}$$

At constant temperature, pressure, and zero work against the external force f ($x = const$), the condition for thermodynamic equilibrium ($dG = 0$) leads to the following expression,

$$\sum_i (\mu_i \nu_i - \mu_i' \nu_i') = 0. \tag{4.30}$$

This is a very important observation. We can associate the first term of this equation with the Gibbs free energy of reagents and the second term with the Gibbs free energy of products, namely,

$$\sum_i \mu_i \nu_i = G_{reagents}, \quad \sum_i \mu_i' \nu_i' = G_{products}. \tag{4.31}$$

The physical meaning of this result is that chemical equilibrium is reached when the chemical potential of the reactants is equal to the chemical potential of products. For more complex systems with many chemical reactions the overall equilibrium is achieved if *all* chemical processes reach the equilibrium as described here.

As we already discussed, chemical potentials cannot be obtained from experiments, so in practice one should use the dependence of the chemical potential on other parameters. Applying the expression for the chemical potential for diluted solutions [see Eq. (4.23)] in Eq. (4.30) will produce the important relation that introduces the chemical *equilibrium constant*, K_{eq},

$$RT \ln K_{eq} = -\Delta G^0, \tag{4.32}$$

with

$$K_{eq} = \frac{\prod c_i^{\prime \nu_i'}}{\prod c_i^{\nu_i}}, \tag{4.33}$$

and

$$\Delta G^0 = \sum_i (\mu_i^{(0)'} \nu_i' - \mu_i^{(0)} \nu_i). \tag{4.34}$$

This quantity is known as a standard Gibbs free energy change for the chemical reaction. The equilibrium constant is the most important qualitative measure of any chemical process. For $K_{eq} > 1$ we have $\Delta G^0 < 0$ and at equilibrium the chemical reaction proceeds forward and the system is dominated by the products. The reaction does not proceed well and the system is mostly filled with reactants for $K_{eq} < 1$ when we have $\Delta G^0 > 0$.

Let us illustrate the importance of equilibrium constant on the example of kinesin motors binding to microtubules. The chemical reaction for this process can be schematically written as

$$K + M = K \cdot M, \tag{4.35}$$

where K labels free kinesin proteins in the solution, M describes microtubules without bound motor proteins, and $K \cdot M$ is for kinesins attached to the cytoskeleton proteins. The equilibrium constant for this reaction can be expressed via concentrations of these species as

$$K_{eq} = \frac{c_{K \cdot M}}{c_K c_M}. \tag{4.36}$$

The physical meaning of this expression is that at constant temperature and pressure, changing the concentration of one of components leads to corresponding modifications of concentrations of other compounds so that the ratio of concentrations, as expressed in Eq. (4.36), remains constant. For example, if we increase the concentration of free kinesins in the solution by a factor of two and keep the concentration of free microtubules the same, to sustain the equilibrium the concentration of motors bound to microtubules will also double.

This theoretical approach also provides a convenient method for analyzing how the external forces can modify the chemical equilibrium, which is relevant for motor protein systems. Let us assume that the reaction in Eq. (4.24) also involves the work against the external constant force f so that after the completion of the reaction the work $f * x_0$ is done. We can connect the variable x in Eq. (4.29) to the chemical variable ξ as

$$x = x_0 \xi. \tag{4.37}$$

This expression can be understood in the following way. When the reaction does not proceed ($\xi = 0$) no work can be done, while for the completion of the chemical transformation ($\xi = 1$) is associated with the work $f * x_0$. Then the condition for the chemical equilibrium ($dG = 0$) at constant temperature and pressure from Eq. (4.29) yields

$$f x_0 + \sum_i (\mu_i \nu_i - \mu_i' \nu_i') = 0. \tag{4.38}$$

It leads to the following force-dependent equilibrium constant, $K_{eq}(f)$,

$$K_{eq}(f) = K_{eq}(f = 0) \exp\left(-\frac{f x_0}{RT}\right). \tag{4.39}$$

One can see that for this system the work against the external force shifts the equilibrium in the backward direction. This result is due to the force-distance work increasing the Gibbs free energy of products, which favors more reactants over the products. For example, let us consider kinesin motor proteins that can make $x_0 = 8$ nm steps against the external forces up to $f = 7$ pN. Each motor molecule does a work equal to $5.6 * 10^{-20}$ J, and a mole of these molecules ($N_A = 6.02 * 10^{23}$) does 33.7 kJ work. At room temperature ($T = 300$ K), we have that $RT \simeq 2.5$ kJ. Then the decrease in the equilibrium constant at room temperature due to the external force is close to 10^6! This is a very significant effect. The important conclusion here is that motor proteins would not be able to proceed forward during cytoskeleton transport if they would function at equilibrium. The constant source of energy supplied by the hydrolysis of ATP or related processes allows molecular motors to work productively in the cellular environment.

4.3 BASIC STATISTICAL MECHANICS

Equilibrium thermodynamics provides a description of macroscopic properties of systems. But the systems that we analyze in physics, chemistry, and biology are usually made from a large number of molecules, and these properties should obviously reflect the actions and interactions of individual molecules. *Statistical mechanics* is a science that gives the *microscopic* interpretation of the macroscopic laws of thermodynamics. It allows us to calculate the thermodynamic functions of a system of specific chemical composition if interactions inside of each molecule as well as inter-molecular interactions are known or can be measured. The important thing to realize is that systems have a very large number of molecules. For example, one mole of any compound consists of $\sim 6 * 10^{23}$ molecules. So for practical reasons it is not possible to take into account all microscopic details of molecular motion and interactions. The calculations must be averaged out over many dynamical states of the system. This is the explanation for the word "statistical." This name was suggested by J.W. Gibbs who also made many significant contributions to the development of statistical mechanics.

The central concept of statistical mechanics is a *Boltzmann distribution law*. It states that the probability of finding a system in a state with the energy E is given by

$$Prob(E) \simeq \exp\left(-\frac{E}{k_B T}\right), \qquad (4.40)$$

where T is the absolute temperature of the system and $k_B = 1.38 \times 10^{-23}$ J/K is known as the Boltzmann constant. The major role in deriving and explaining the theoretical framework for statistical mechanics was played by the world-famous Austrian physicist Ludwig Boltzmann who is shown in Fig. 4.3.

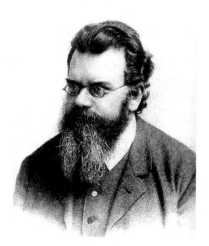

FIGURE 4.3   Ludwig Boltzmann (1844–1906). The famous Austrian physicist who developed the foundations and the mathematical apparatus of statistical mechanics.

The exponential form of the Boltzmann distribution law can be understood using the observation that the probability of two independent events is a product of probabilities for each event. To explain this, let us analyze a system that in some state has the energy E_1 and in other state it has the energy E_2. We assume also that the occurrences of these two states are independent of each other. For example, consider a system that has one microtubule molecule and two kinesin motor proteins. Let us assume that the first state of the system describes the conditions with one of the motor molecules being free in the solution, and the second state is associated with the motor protein bound to the microtubule. These two states are obviously independent of each other. Let us then view the combined state when one kinesin is in the solution and another one is bound to the microtubule. The energy for this combined state is equal to $E_1 + E_2$. The probability of observing this state should be equal to the product of separate probabilities for the states 1 and 2, because they are independent. So we have the following expression for the probabilities,

$$Prob(E_1 + E_2) = Prob(E_1) * Prob(E_2). \tag{4.41}$$

One can see that the only function that can satisfy this requirement is the exponential function. We have then

$$\exp\left(-\frac{E_1 + E_2}{k_B T}\right) = \exp\left(-\frac{E_1}{k_B T}\right) * \exp\left(-\frac{E_2}{k_B T}\right). \tag{4.42}$$

Note, however, that we could never explain the fact that the coefficient in the exponent is inversely proportional to the temperature. This can be regarded as a basic definition of temperature or, alternatively, as a law of nature.

We can directly apply the Boltzmann distribution law to any macroscopic system where the state i has the energy E_i. Then at equilibrium at the temperature T the probability of finding the system in the specific state i is given by

$$P_i = \frac{\exp\left(-\frac{E_i}{k_B T}\right)}{\sum_i \exp\left(-\frac{E_i}{k_B T}\right)}. \tag{4.43}$$

This is the consequence of the fact that the sum of all probabilities should be equal to one, i.e., the normalization condition. This is an important result because it allows us to connect the microscopic features of molecules with thermodynamic functions of the system, which is the main goal of statistical mechanics. Thermodynamic functions can be viewed as properties that are averaged over different states of the system.

The next step is to identify the thermodynamic internal energy U as a mean energy of the system, $< E > \equiv U$. That average energy at constant temperature can be easily calculated via the Boltzmann distribution,

$$< E > = \frac{\sum_i E_i \exp\left(-\frac{E_i}{k_B T}\right)}{\sum_i \exp\left(-\frac{E_i}{k_B T}\right)}. \tag{4.44}$$

The connection of U with the microscopic properties can be seen using the following arguments. The energy levels E_i of the system depend on the volume, V, temperature, T, and the chemical composition, i.e., on the number of molecules $N_1, N_2, \ldots$ of each of chemical species that are present in the system. The energy of each state is a sum of energies of individual molecules.

We can rewrite Eq. (4.44) as,

$$U = <E> = - \left[\frac{\partial}{\partial \frac{1}{k_B T}} \ln \sum_i \exp \left(-\frac{E_i}{k_B T} \right) \right]_{V, N_1, N_2, \ldots} . \qquad (4.45)$$

It follows from the mathematical identity $(d \ln x / dx) = 1/x$. The argument under the logarithm is defined as a *partition function* Z,

$$Z = \sum_i \exp \left(-\frac{E_i}{k_B T} \right). \qquad (4.46)$$

Then the internal energy can also be written in the following concise form

$$U = k_B T^2 \left(\frac{\partial \ln Z}{\partial T} \right)_{V, N_1, N_2, \ldots} . \qquad (4.47)$$

The partition function Z is a central quantity in statistical mechanics because *all* thermodynamic functions can be evaluated utilizing this function. For example, using the relations between various thermodynamic functions one can show that the Helmholtz free energy can be expressed as

$$F = -k_B T \ln Z. \qquad (4.48)$$

This is the most important equation in statistical mechanics. Applying the equality $S = (U - F)/T$ we can obtain the connection between the entropy and the partition function,

$$S = \frac{U}{T} + k_B \ln Z. \qquad (4.49)$$

It can be shown that the pressure can be also expressed in the simple form in terms of the partition function,

$$P = k_B T \left(\frac{\partial \ln Z}{\partial V} \right)_{T, N_1, N_2, \ldots} . \qquad (4.50)$$

The statistical analog for the Gibbs free energy is given by

$$G = -k_B T \ln Z + k_B T \left(\frac{\partial \ln Z}{\partial \ln V} \right)_{T, N_1, N_2, \ldots} . \qquad (4.51)$$

We conclude that all thermodynamic parameters can be calculated in terms of the partition function Z or its derivatives. Sometimes, there is no need even to know Z explicitly, but only its dependence on some variables $(T, V, \ldots)$ is required. For example, as one can see from Eq. (4.50), to compute pressure it will be enough to have the information of the dependence of the partition function on V.

One of the greatest successes of statistical mechanics is the ability to present a microscopic explanation for the entropy. Boltzmann derived the most celebrated equation in statistical mechanics,

$$S = k_B \ln W, \qquad (4.52)$$

where W might be interpreted as the total number of states at specific values of the internal energy U, number of particles in the system N, and the volume of the system V. The entropy is just a logarithmic measure of this number.

Thus, the prescription of the statistical mechanics for calculating thermodynamic functions of the system is the following. From information on molecular properties one can estimate the energy of all possible states of the system, which will lead to the expression for the partition function. The knowledge of Z then provides the connections with thermodynamic parameters, as described above.

4.4 APPLICATION FOR MOTOR PROTEINS

Equilibrium thermodynamics and statistical mechanics provide a comprehensive fundamental framework for explaining all properties of any system. However, the analysis can only be applied for systems that reach equilibrium. It is known that all biological processes are strongly in non-equilibrium, and this significantly limits the application of thermodynamics and statistical mechanics for biological molecular motors. There is a flow of energy into and out of motor proteins, and one cannot apply equilibrium approaches in determining their properties. In addition, equilibrium thermodynamics and statistical mechanics do not discuss how properties of molecules change with the time. But the dynamic aspect is very important for understanding mechanisms of motor proteins.

Although the application of methods of equilibrium thermodynamics and statistical mechanics for motor proteins might be limited, one should remember that the introduced fundamental concepts still allow us to obtain significant input on the functioning of these systems. First, some chemical and physical processes in motor protein systems can be viewed as in local equilibrium, at least, for some periods of time. Furthermore, one has to use the Gibbs free energy to describe any process associated with biological molecular motors. The process will proceed if it is thermodynamically favorable, i.e., if the free energy is going down. Thermodynamics also provides important bounds for various properties of motor proteins. For example, if thermodynamic calculations suggest that a given process is unfavorable, then we can argue that most probably it will not occur. This will help to eliminate mechanisms that are not thermodynamically consistent. In addition, the known amount of free energy released during the hydrolysis of ATP or related processes gives the upper bound of possible work that motor proteins can do against the external loads during each enzymatic cycle. This will also limit the range of possible dynamic mechanisms for molecular motors. Specific applications of fundamental concepts from equilibrium thermodynamics and statistical mechanics for various motor proteins will be given in future chapters.

4.5 SUMMARY

In this chapter we started the discussion of theoretical concepts and fundamental ideas that are needed for understanding mechanisms of biological molecular motors. It was argued that because motor proteins are involved in heat transformations and also participate in multiple chemical reactions, one should explore the ideas of equilibrium thermodynamics and statistical mechanics. We presented a brief review of basic concepts of equilibrium thermodynamics. It was argued that any system can be described by various thermodynamic functions that can be viewed as macroscopic properties of these systems. The most important function for analyzing various processes in chemistry, physics, and biology is the Gibbs free energy. At a given temperature and pressure, a process will go forward if it is associated with lowering of the free energy. To analyze chemical reactions, one should employ the related concept of the chemical potential. It was shown that the equilibrium in chemical reactions is achieved when the chemical potential of reactants becomes equal to the chemical potential of products. The most important parameter to describe the chemical equilibrium is the equilibrium constant. We also discussed how the external forces might shift the chemical equilibrium, which must be relevant for motor proteins that function in cells against a variety of loads and barriers.

To connect thermodynamic functions of systems with microscopic properties, we introduced basic ideas from statistical mechanics. The key concept of statistical mechanics is the Boltzmann distribution law which specifies the probability of observing specific states of the system. It was argued that all thermodynamic parameters can be calculated explicitly if one can determine the partition function from the molecular properties.

Finally, we discussed the application of ideas from equilibrium thermodynamics and statistical mechanics for motor protein systems. However, these ideas have a limited use because biological molecular motors function under non-equilibrium conditions. At the same time, equilibrium thermodynamics and statistical mechanics are still useful in analyzing various processes associated with motor proteins. They help specifically by eliminating possible mechanisms that contradict thermodynamics.

CHAPTER 5

Fundamental Physical Concepts: Non-Equilibrium Approaches

CONTENTS

5.1 INTRODUCTION

Our efforts to explain the mechanisms of motor proteins must take into account the fact that their properties are not constant but evolve in time and might fluctuate. Motor proteins can bind to their cellular tracks (nucleic acids or cytoskeleton filaments), or dissociate from them. They could also collide with other molecules in the cytosol and even stick for some time to other cellular objects. During the chemical processes when motor proteins function as enzymes, they go through a variety of molecular conformations and biochemical states, and this behavior is repeated many times. This complex dynamics is critical for understanding biological molecular motors. However, equilibrium thermodynamics always assumes that any system is in equilibrium, i.e., no changes in properties of molecules are observed with time. Statistical mechanics allows us to calculate macroscopic features of systems from molecular properties, but it can be done only for equilibrium systems. Both of these fundamental approaches neglect the time-dependent features of motor proteins. At the same time, we know that motor proteins in cells operate at non-equilibrium conditions, i.e., their properties might change with time. For example, at one time the motor protein might be bound to the filaments transporting the cellular cargo, while at another time it became inactive after dissociating from the track. It is important to understand this temporal evolution at the single-molecule level.

More specifically we are interested in answering the following questions concerning the microscopic functioning of motor proteins in the cellular environment:

1. How are dynamic properties of motor proteins such as velocities, dispersions, and exerted forces related to chemical transition rates at the molecular level?

2. What is the coupling between hydrolysis or other enzymatically supported processes and mechanical transformations in biological molecular motors?

3. How do the external forces modify dynamic properties of motor proteins and what can this tell us about mechanisms of functioning of biological motors?

4. How can we understand the information from single-molecule experiments on residence times of motor proteins at various spatial positions? In what way is this coupled with chemical states of biological motors?

To investigate times and rates of chemical reactions and processes that are taking place in motor protein systems, we will use various methods of *chemical kinetics*. The connections between molecular transitions and macroscopic dynamic properties of biological motors will be investigated using the concepts of *random walks*. The analysis of stepping transitions and residence times will be done using the concepts of *first-passage processes*.

5.2 MACROSCOPIC CHEMICAL KINETICS

It was observed by chemists long ago that during chemical reactions concentrations of reactants and products vary with time. Probably, the first quantitative experimental study of a chemical reaction was done by a German scientist Ludwig Ferdinand Wilhelmy in 1850 (Wilhelmy 1850) [182]. He investigated the acid-catalyzed conversion of sucrose into a mixture of fructose and glucose by using the polarimetry technique. Wilhelmy found that the rate of this reaction was proportional to the amounts of sugar and acid, and also depended on the temperature. Unfortunately, this work was not appreciated by contemporary scientists; its importance become clear only 30–40 years later.

Generally, in chemical reactions, one can observe that the concentrations of reactants decrease, while the concentrations of products increase with time (Houston 2001) [67]. Fig. 3.1A in this book shows the example of changes in the concentration of ADP during the action of Ncd motor proteins that hydrolyze ATP molecules. In this case, ADP molecules are products and their amount is growing with time. These variations in quantities of participants of chemical reactions can be monitored quite precisely by various experimental techniques, including spectroscopic, electrochemical, and volumetric methods (Houston 2001) [67].

To make the description of chemical reactions more quantitative, consider a general chemical reaction that can be represented by the following stoichiometric equation,

$$aA + bB \rightleftharpoons cC + dD. \tag{5.1}$$

This states that a molecules of type A react with b molecules of type B to create c molecules of type C and d molecules of type D. The rate of this chemical reaction R is defined in the following way,

$$R = \frac{1}{c}\frac{d[C]}{dt} = \frac{1}{d}\frac{d[D]}{dt} = -\frac{1}{a}\frac{d[A]}{dt} = -\frac{1}{b}\frac{d[B]}{dt}, \tag{5.2}$$

where $[A]$ is the concentration of species A, etc. Note that because the changes in concentrations of all molecules are not independent of each other, as suggested by the stoichiometry in Eq. (5.1), the temporal evolution of this reaction can be conveniently estimated by monitoring the change in the concentration of only one component. It is natural to assume that the rate of this chemical reaction is a function of the concentrations of participating chemicals,

$$R = f([A], [B], [C], [D]). \tag{5.3}$$

This expression is known as a *rate law* (Houston 2001, Steinfeld et al. 1999) [67, 155]. The goal of macroscopic or phenomenological chemical kinetics is to determine this function explicitly. Then the changes of concentrations of molecules in the system with time can be fully evaluated.

In general, the rate law is an unknown function. However, based on large numbers of empirical observations of various chemical processes, it can often be written as a product expression of the form (Houston 2001, Steinfeld et al. 1999) [67, 155],

$$R = k[A]^m[B]^n[C]^o[D]^p, \tag{5.4}$$

where the coefficient k is known as the *rate constant* while parameters m, n, o and p may be nonnegative numbers. The sum of these parameters defines the *overall order* of the chemical reaction,

$$q = m + n + o + p. \tag{5.5}$$

The important observation here is that the order of the reaction might not be related with the stoichiometry of the process given in Eq. (5.1). This is because Eq.(5.1) is a macroscopic equation, i.e., it is a result of combining several elementary chemical transitions. This specific set of elementary processes is known as the mechanism of this chemical reaction. The order of the reaction obviously depends on details of the mechanism.

5.2.1 Irreversible Processes

The idea behind the order of the reaction is that different orders correspond to different microscopic mechanisms of chemical reactions. To illustrate this, we consider first the simplest *first-order* reactions of the general type $A \to P$, where P stands for products. The differential form of the rate law for this process can be written as

$$R = \frac{d[A]}{dt} = -k[A]. \tag{5.6}$$

The sign "minus" in this expression reflects the fact that the concentration of molecules A is decreasing during the reaction. This differential equation can be easily solved if we first rearrange it as

$$\frac{d[A]}{[A]} = -kdt. \tag{5.7}$$

Integrating this equation from time $t = 0$ to t leads to a relation that describes the temporal evolution of the concentration of the reactant molecules A,

$$[A](t) = A_0 \exp(-kt), \tag{5.8}$$

where $A_0 = [A](t = 0)$. This expression is also known as an integral form of the rate law. Thus, in first-order chemical reactions the concentration of the reactant is exponentially decaying with an exponent proportional to the rate constant k, as shown in Fig. 5.1. In experiments, to test the investigated process one should plot $\ln[A]$ as a function of time. If a linear dependence is observed, then the process is most probably a first-order chemical reaction, as suggested by Eq. (5.8).

There are two natural time scales in the first-order chemical reaction, and both of them are frequently used in analyzing experiments (Houston 2001) [67]. The *half-life* of the reactant, $\tau_{1/2}$, is defined as a time at which the concentration decreases to $1/2$ of its original value. From Eq. (5.8) it can be shown that

$$\tau_{1/2} = \frac{\ln 2}{k}. \tag{5.9}$$

Interestingly, this time does not depend on the original concentration A_0. A different time scale, called the *lifetime*, $\tau = 1/k$, defines the time when the concentration is lower by a factor of e. Both of these time scales are indicated in Fig. 5.1.

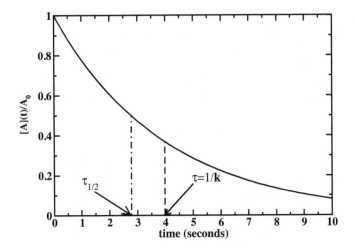

FIGURE 5.1 A normalized concentration profile for a reactant compound in the first-order chemical reaction with rate constant $k = 0.25$ s^{-1}; see Eq. (5.8). The half-life of the reactant is marked at $\tau_{1/2}$, while the lifetime of the reactant is at $\tau = 1/k$.

Second-order chemical reactions can be generally written as

$$A + B \to P. \tag{5.10}$$

How concentrations evolve in time for this case is derived in the Mathematical Appendix. Here we analyze a simpler case with all reactants being of the same type, i.e., $2A \to P$. The differential rate law is then given by

$$R = -\frac{1}{2}\frac{d[A]}{dt} = k[A]^2. \tag{5.11}$$

Initially, we had only molecules of type A and $A_0 = [A](t = 0)$. This expression can be rearranged to obtain

$$\frac{d[A]}{[A]^2} = -2kdt. \tag{5.12}$$

Integrating left and right sides of this equation from $t = 0$ up to the time t leads to

$$\frac{1}{[A](t)} - \frac{1}{A_0} = 2kt. \tag{5.13}$$

This suggests that a second-order reaction is observed if experiments indicate that the inverse concentrations are proportional to the time. For the second-order reaction again we can define the half-life, $\tau_{1/2}$, for which from Eq. (5.13) one can obtain

$$\tau_{1/2} = \frac{1}{2kA_0}. \tag{5.14}$$

The important observation here is that the half-life, in contrast to the first-order processes, depends on the initial concentration of the reactant. This might be another way of distinguishing first-order reactions from second-order processes in experiments.

One can generalize this analysis for an n-th order chemical reaction with the same type of reactant, i.e., $nA \rightarrow P$. For this process the reaction rate is given by

$$R = -\frac{1}{n}\frac{d[A]}{dt} = k[A]^n, \qquad (5.15)$$

which can be solved by direct integration, as we did for the first-order and second-order processes. This produces the following relation on temporal evolution of the concentration of the reactant A,

$$\frac{1}{(n-1)[A]^{n-1}(t)} - \frac{1}{(n-1)A_0^{n-1}} = nkt. \qquad (5.16)$$

As expected, for $n = 2$ it reduces to Eq. (5.13). In experimental studies, one might conclude that the n-th order process is observed if the quantity $[A]^{-(n-1)}$ becomes proportional to the time.

Let us consider a more complex system where two parallel chemical reactions are taking place,

$$A \rightarrow B \qquad (5.17)$$

with the rate constant k_1; and

$$A \rightarrow C \qquad (5.18)$$

with the rate constant k_2. The temporal evolution of concentrations of compounds A, B, and C in this system can be described by a set of differential equations,

$$\frac{d[A]}{dt} = -(k_1 + k_2)[A], \qquad (5.19)$$

$$\frac{d[B]}{dt} = k_1[A], \quad \frac{d[C]}{dt} = k_1[A]. \qquad (5.20)$$

Again, we assume that at $t = 0$ we have only molecules of type A with the initial concentration A_0. The first of these equations is identical to the first-order chemical reaction with an effective rate constant given by the sum $k_1 + k_2$. So we can easily write the solution as

$$[A](t) = A_0 \exp[-(k_1 + k_2)t]. \qquad (5.21)$$

Substituting this result into Eqs. (5.21) leads to

$$\frac{d[B]}{dt} = k_1 A_0 \exp[-(k_1 + k_2)t], \qquad (5.22)$$

$$\frac{d[C]}{dt} = k_2 A_0 \exp[-(k_1 + k_2)t]. \tag{5.23}$$

Integrating these equations and taking into account the fact that at $t = 0$ there were no products, we obtain the final expressions for the growth with time of the concentrations of B and C,

$$[B] = \frac{k_1}{k_1 + k_2} A_0 (1 - \exp[-(k_1 + k_2)t]), \tag{5.24}$$

$$[C] = \frac{k_2}{k_1 + k_2} A_0 (1 - \exp[-(k_1 + k_2)t]). \tag{5.25}$$

This system can be conveniently analyzed by looking into a *branching ratio*, r, which describes the ratio of concentrations of products,

$$r = \frac{[B](t)}{[C](t)} = \frac{k_1}{k_2}. \tag{5.26}$$

There are two interesting observations about such parallel chemical reactions. First, the branching ratio is time independent. Second, Eqs. (5.24) and (5.25) suggest that the characteristic times for approaching to the final values of the concentrations for *both* products are given by $\tau = 1/(k_1 + k_2)$. This contrasts with naive expectations for the times to be equal $1/k_1$ and $1/k_2$. The reason is that the rates of creating product molecules are proportional to the concentration of A, although with different coefficients of proportionality. But the concentration $[A]$ decays with the effective rate constant equal to $k_{eff} = k_1 + k_2$. This example shows that it might be dangerous to consider specific chemical reactions separately from other processes in systems where many reactions are taking place simultaneously. This might be relevant for motor protein systems.

Another important system for understanding the methods of chemical kinetics is two consecutive chemical reactions (Houston 2001) [67], such as

$$A \rightarrow B \rightarrow C. \tag{5.27}$$

Here we assume that the first reaction $(A \rightarrow B)$ is taking place with rate constant k_1, while the second step $(B \rightarrow C)$ is described by the rate constant k_2. For this system the concentrations of all compounds vary in time according to the following chemical kinetic equations:

$$\frac{d[A]}{dt} = -k_1[A], \tag{5.28}$$

$$\frac{d[B]}{dt} = k_1[A] - k_2[B], \tag{5.29}$$

$$\frac{d[C]}{dt} = k_2[B]. \tag{5.30}$$

If we also assume that initially only molecules of type A are in the system with the concentration A_0, then the temporal evolution of A molecules can be easily obtained. It is simply a first-order reaction, and as we argued above, it yields

$$[A](t) = A_0 \exp(-k_1 t). \tag{5.31}$$

Substituting this result into Eq. (5.29) leads to an explicit expression for the temporal evolution of B molecules (Houston 2001) [67], namely,

$$[B](t) = \frac{k_1}{k_2 - k_1} A_0 \left[\exp(-k_1 t) - \exp(-k_2 t) \right]. \tag{5.32}$$

Finally, the concentration of C molecules can be easily obtained from the following arguments. The total number of molecules of all types in this system is constant, as suggested by Eq. (5.27). One can see that when one molecule of A reacts we produce exactly one molecule of B, and the total number of molecules does not change. If one B molecule disappears it is always associated with the appearance of one C molecule. This is known as a *mass balance condition*. Thus, we have

$$[C](t) = A_0 - [A](t) - [B](t). \tag{5.33}$$

The time-dependent concentrations of molecules A, B, and C are shown in Fig. 5.2.

The set of sequential chemical reactions is a convenient system for introducing one of the most successful methods in chemical kinetics for calculating concentration profiles and chemical rates. It is called a *steady-state approximation* (SSA). To illustrate this approach let us assume that molecules B are very reactive, i.e., $k_2 \gg k_1$. From Eq. (5.32) we obtain that

$$[B](t) \simeq \frac{k_1}{k_2} A_0 \exp(-k_1 t) = \frac{k_1}{k_2} [A](t). \tag{5.34}$$

It suggests that $k_2 [B](t) \simeq k_1 [A](t)$ which, after employing Eq. (5.30), leads to a conclusion that $\frac{d[B]}{dt} \simeq 0$. Note from Fig. 5.2 (where $k_2/k_1 = 10$) that the concentration of B molecules after some initial period ($\simeq 1$ s) goes into a regime where it changes very slowly, in agreement with our arguments. The physical meaning of this statement is that highly reactive intermediate molecules quickly reach steady-state conditions when their concentrations do not change much with time. This is a reason for the name of the SSA method. One can also see that SSA provides a significant simplification for calculating chemical kinetic properties: instead of solving differential equations, one may solve much simpler algebraic equations.

5.2.2 *Reversible Processes*

All chemical reactions considered so far are irreversible, i.e., the reactions will not stop until all reactants are consumed. Chemical equilibrium in such systems cannot be established. Although there are processes that can be viewed

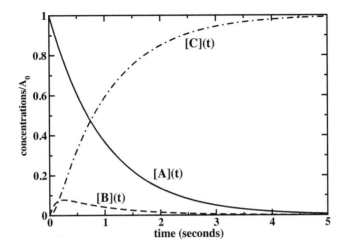

FIGURE 5.2 Normalized concentration profiles for the molecules A, B, and C in the sequential chemical reaction given by Eq. (5.27) with the rate constant $k_1 = 1 \ s^{-1}$ and $k_2 = 1 \ s^{-1}$.

as irreversible, at least for some periods of time, an overwhelming majority of chemical reactions in biological systems, including motor proteins, are reversible. So it is more realistic to analyze the simplest reversible chemical reaction such as

$$A \rightleftharpoons B. \qquad (5.35)$$

Here we assume that k_1 and k_{-1} are rate constants for the forward and backward transitions, respectively. The rate of the overall chemical reaction can be written as

$$R = \frac{d[B]}{dt} = k_1[A] - k_{-1}[B]. \qquad (5.36)$$

It is assumed that initial concentrations of molecules A and B are equal to A_0 and B_0, respectively. If we wait for long times, the system will reach an equilibrium state in which the decay of A molecules is fully compensated by a creation from B molecules. Let us define A_e and B_e as equilibrium concentrations for molecules A and B. At equilibrium the rate of chemical reaction is equal to zero because two opposing processes balance each other. In mathematical terms from Eq. (5.36) it means that

$$k_1 A_{eq} = k_{-1} B_{eq}. \qquad (5.37)$$

One could also define an equilibrium constant for this process, which following our discussions on chemical equilibrium in Chapter 4—see Eq. (4.32)—can be written as

$$K_{eq} = \frac{B_{eq}}{A_{eq}}. \qquad (5.38)$$

Then it leads us to a very important result,

$$K_{eq} = \frac{k_1}{k_{-1}}. \tag{5.39}$$

This equation expresses the fact that the equilibrium constant is equal to the ratio of forward and backward rate constants. This provides a connection between thermodynamic properties (equilibrium constants) and chemical kinetic parameters (rate constants). This fundamental statement is frequently associated with the *principle of detailed balance*. In complex systems with many processes the overall equilibrium is achieved only when all elementary chemical step rates in opposite directions balance each other (Berry et al. 2002) [20]. This principle was first formulated by Boltzmann for kinetic studies of molecular collisions.

For the system of opposing chemical reactions, one may also evaluate how concentrations of all molecules change with time. The details of such calculations are given in the Mathematical Appendix. Here we just present the results:

$$[A](t) = A_e + (A_0 - A_e)e^{-(k_1+k_{-1})t}, \tag{5.40}$$

$$[B](t) = B_e + (B_0 - B_e)e^{-(k_1+k_{-1})t}. \tag{5.41}$$

One can see that the approach to the equilibrium is associated with a time scale $\tau = 1/(k_1 + k_{-1})$. This result is significant since it shows that concentrations of both molecules in the reversible chemical reactions depend on the sum of forward and backward rates. Again, it does not agree with naive expectations that one could draw erroneously from just looking separately at forward and backward chemical reactions.

5.2.3 *Temperature Dependence*

One of the most striking properties of chemical reactions is their strong dependence on temperature. From our everyday experience we know that heating strongly accelerates many chemical reactions. For example, paper is very stable in air at room temperature, but after igniting the piece of paper it will quickly burn. In 1889, Swedish scientist Svante Arrhenius (see Fig. 5.3) proposed that rate constants for all chemical processes follow the empirical relationship,

$$k = A \exp\left(-\frac{E_a}{RT}\right), \tag{5.42}$$

where the pre-exponential factor A does not depend on T while E_a is called the *activation energy*, and $R = 8.31$ J/K is a molar gas constant. This relation is known now as the *Arrhenius Law*.

The Arrhenius Law is one of the most important results in chemical kinetics since it allows one to obtain a significant amount of the information on the mechanisms of underlying chemical processes. It argues that during

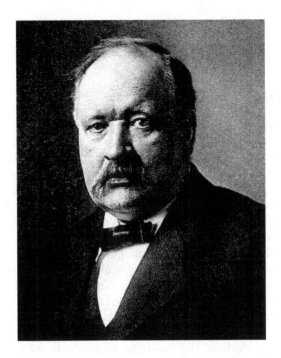

FIGURE 5.3 The famous Swedish physical chemist Svante Arrhenius (1859–1927) who is one of the founders of modern chemical kinetics. It is interesting that although Svante Arrhenius made several fundamental contributions to chemistry he was almost forced to leave the field of chemistry. As an undergraduate student he was not very successful, and his PhD. work on electrolytes was poorly evaluated. Ironically, for the same work he received a Nobel Prize in chemistry in 1903.

any chemical reaction some energy barrier should be overcome [see E_a in Eq. (5.42)]. Then the higher the temperature, the easier it is for molecules to pass this activation barrier. Another interpretation of the temperature dependence given by the Arrhenius Law is the fact that at the microscopic level, reactions are taking place as a result of molecular collisions that have enough energy. Increasing the temperature makes these collisions more frequent, leading to faster chemical reactions. From an experimental point of view, the Arrhenius behavior is observed if the logarithm of the rate constant is proportional to the inverse temperature,

$$\ln k = \ln A - \frac{E_a}{RT},\tag{5.43}$$

as one can see from Eq. (5.42).

It is also important to note here that many systems do not follow the simple Arrhenius Law. This usually means that the mechanisms needed to explain such behavior cannot be viewed as overcoming a single energy barrier. For example, it might involve many coupled chemical processes with comparable activation barriers so that there is no clear rate-limiting step under the given experimental conditions.

5.3 RANDOM WALKS

In our discussion of activities of motor proteins in cells we frequently used the analogy with a large city. We argued that the motion of biological molecular motors along the cytoskeleton filaments and nucleic acids looks similar to cars driving along the streets and highways. This is a very useful analogy. However, the details of the motion of cars and trucks are very different from motor proteins. Cars drive along the roads with usually high speeds without significant variations. They stop only at intersections or at stop signs or if they encounter traffic. This kind of motion can be called *ballistic* or deterministic. But the details of the motor proteins' dynamics in cells are very different. If we could focus on a single motor, we would see that the protein stays at the specific location of the filament for some time, then it jumps forward. After this it sits again at another spacial location for some time and then it moves again. This process repeats many times. The time periods between jumps seem to be random, i.e., these time intervals are not the same but follow some broad distribution. In addition, the molecular motor molecule can sometimes step backward or even dissociate completely from the filament track. This type of random dynamics is called *stochastic*. To better understand the nature of motor protein motions it is very useful to introduce the concept of *random walks*. This is the idea of how to describe the random motion of any object, and it has found multiple successful applications in chemistry, physics, biology as well as in economics, ecology, psychology, and social sciences (van Kampen 2001, Rudnick and Gaspari 2004) [174, 136].

Let us consider a simple example of the random walk where a particle, which we also call a walker, can hop on a one-dimensional lattice as shown in Fig. 5.4. At $t = 0$ the random walker starts at the origin. It can jump one site to the right with a probability p, or with a probability $q = 1 - p$ it can hop to the left neighboring site. We assume that the random walk does not have memory, i.e., each event (to jump to the right or to the left) is independent of what happened before. This is similar to a situation when the direction of the motion is decided every time by flipping a coin. In the case of coin flipping, we have $p = q = 1/2$, and the random walk is the unbiased symmetric process. The random walker with equal probability can step in either direction. We consider a more general case of a biased asymmetric process with $p \neq q$. This situation might better describe biological molecular motors, which generally have a preferential direction for their motion.

Now let us suppose that the random walker made N steps, and some of them were to the right and some were to the left, but the walker ends up at the position m. The range of possible values for m is from $-N$ to N. We define n_r as a number of steps that the random walker made in the forward

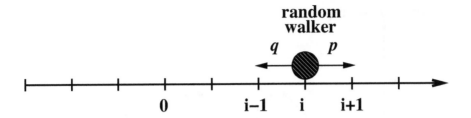

FIGURE 5.4 A schematic view of a random walker moving along a one-dimensional lattice. The particle at site i can jump with a probability p to the site $i+1$ or with a probability q to the site $i-1$. At the initial time $t=0$ the random walker started at the origin $i=0$.

(right direction), and correspondingly, n_l describes the number of steps to the left. Obviously, we have

$$N = n_r + n_l. \tag{5.44}$$

This also allows us to determine the final position m,

$$m = n_r - n_l. \tag{5.45}$$

There are many possibilities for the random walker during these N steps. For illustration, let us view the case of only $N = 3$ steps, as illustrated in Fig. 5.5. Then there are four possible outcomes of where the random walker will be found after three steps. Here we assume that the step size is equal to one. The random walker can make three steps to the right ($n_r = 3$ and $n_l = 0$) and it will end up at the position $m = 3$. The random walker can make two steps to the right and one to the left ($n_r = 2$ and $n_l = 1$), and its final position will be at $m = 1$. Similarly, for two steps to the left and one to the right ($n_r = 1$ and $n_l = 2$) the walker will arrive at $m = -1$. For all steps to the left ($n_r = 0$ and $n_l = 3$) its final position will be at $m = -3$. In addition, there might be more than one way for the random walker to reach the final site m. For example, for $m = 1$ there are three different trajectories that lead to the same final position. If we assign $+1$ to the right step and -1 to the left step, then these trajectories might be graphically expressed as $(-1, +1, +1)$, $(+1, -1, +1)$, and $(+1, +1, -1)$. It means that in the first trajectory the random walker first steps to the left and then makes two right jumps. In the second trajectory it first steps to the right, then moves backward and after this again steps to the right. In the third trajectory there are two hoppings to the right that are followed by a step to the left.

For a general random walk we are interested in a question of how to estimate a probability $P_N(m)$ to find the random walker at the position m after N steps if it started from $i = 0$. To calculate this quantity we need to determine the number of the random walk trajectories that end at m, and dividing

number of steps

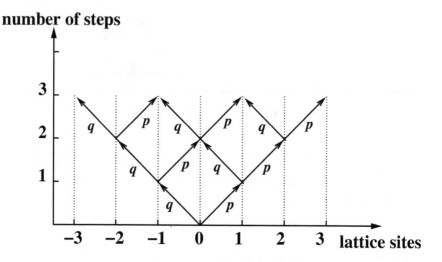

FIGURE 5.5 An illustrative example of the random walk trajectories after $N = 3$ steps. The forward steps have the probability p, while the probability for the backward steps is q.

this over the total number of trajectories with N steps will lead us to the answer. In other words, the probability of trajectories that finish at the site m must be evaluated. A specific trajectory consisting of n_r steps to the right and n_l steps to the left has a probability $p^{n_r} * q^{n_l}$ since each event is independent of each other. But there are several trajectories that have the same n_r and n_s. These arguments suggest the following estimate of the probability of trajectories with fixed n_r and n_l,

$$P_N(m) = C_{n_r}^N p^{n_r} * q^{n_l}, \qquad (5.46)$$

where the parameter $C_{n_r}^N$ is known as a binomial coefficient and it is given by

$$C_{n_r}^N = \frac{N!}{(n_r!)(n_l!)}, \qquad (5.47)$$

and we also remind the reader that $n_r = N - n_l$. This equation can be understood by explicitly counting trajectories. We are interested in all trajectories with fixed n_r and n_s values, which are independent of the sequence of the right and left steps. So the order of these jumps can be switched, and because there is a total of N steps we have a factor of $N!$ of different trajectories that one might obtain by performing this procedure for all steps. But this argument overestimates the correct number of trajectories with fixed n_r and n_l because if we switch between jumps of two right steps or two left steps, we do not get new trajectories. Steps in the same direction are indistinguishable! Different trajectories are obtained only if we switch left and right steps. To correct for this overcounting we must divide by $(n_r!)(n_l!)$. Then we come to the expression given in Eq. (5.46). The number of right and left steps can be expressed in terms of N and m from Eqs. (5.44) and (5.45), producing

$$n_r = \frac{1}{2}(N+m), \quad n_l = \frac{1}{2}(N-m). \tag{5.48}$$

Finally, the probability for the random walker to reach the site m after N steps is given by

$$P_N(m) = \frac{N!}{[(N+m)/2]!([(N-m)/2]!)} p^{\frac{N+m}{2}} * (1-p)^{\frac{N-m}{2}}. \tag{5.49}$$

To illustrate these calculations we plot this function in Fig. 5.6 for the random walk with $p = 0.8$. More specifically, the probability of reaching a position m for $N = 10$ steps is presented. Because the random walker prefers to jump to the right, the most probable positions are much closer to the $m = 10$ than to the $m = -10$ limit, as one would expect. The most probable position corresponds to $m = 7$ for this set of parameters.

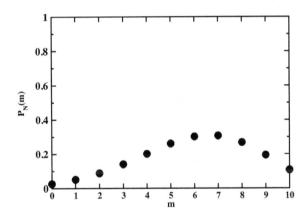

FIGURE 5.6 The probability for the random walker to be found at the site m after $N = 10$ steps when $p = 0.8$. Note that there is also a non-zero probability for the random walk to be found at $m < 0$ sites, but it is very small and we do not show it.

The function $P_N(m)$ is a central quantity for analysis of a random walk since it allows us to calculate all properties of the system. For example, if one is interested in determining of the average position of the random walker, say $\langle m \rangle$, for the total number of N steps, it can be found from

$$\langle m \rangle = \sum_{m=-N}^{N} m P_N(m). \tag{5.50}$$

The detailed calculations presented in the Mathematical Appendix show that the expression for the average position is quite simple,

$$\langle m \rangle = N(p-q) = N(2p-1). \tag{5.51}$$

This result is intuitively very clear. We expect that the average number of the right steps to be equal to Np and the average number of the left steps is expected to be Nq. For parameters employed in Fig. 5.6 ($N = 10$ and $p = 0.8$) we obtain $\langle m \rangle = 6$, which agrees reasonably well with naive estimates that one could make by just looking at the plot of $P_N(m)$. The reason that the average value is slightly lower than the maximal value in the distribution function $P_N(m)$ is the asymmetry of this probability function. It means that there is a small but non-negligible contribution of small m values that lowers the average value in comparison with the most probable position. More involved calculations are needed to compute other moments of the motion of the random walker. For the second moment in the random walker position it can be shown that

$$\langle m^2 \rangle = 4Npq + N^2(p-q)^2. \tag{5.52}$$

Another important quantity to characterize the random walker is a variance in the position which is defined as

$$\sigma^2(m) = \langle m^2 \rangle - \langle m \rangle^2. \tag{5.53}$$

It is related to the width of the distribution of the probability function $P_N(m)$ (see Fig. 5.6) and it qualitatively describes a measure of the "randomness" for the random walker. The larger this parameter, the more random the dynamics of the random walker, i.e., it changes the direction of the motion more frequently. The smaller the variance, the less stochastic the motion of the walker, approaching the ballistic regime (like cars on highways). Using Eqs. (5.51) and (5.52), we obtain that the variance in the position of the random walker is given by

$$\sigma^2(m) = 4Npq = 4Np(1-p). \tag{5.54}$$

It is interesting to analyze this result. The largest variation is found for the unbiased random walk with $p = 1/2$. In this case, the random walker at average switches the direction of the motion at each jump. At the same time, the ballistic motion is realized for $p = 1$ or $p = 0$ when the random walker does not change the direction of the motion.

There is a different way of analyzing properties of the random walk. We can write the following equation,

$$P_{N+1}(m) = pP_N(m-1) + qP_N(m+1) + (1-p-q)P_N(m). \tag{5.55}$$

This relation reflects the fact that the site m can be reached from the neighboring site $m-1$ with the probability p or from the site $m+1$ with the probability q. In addition, we assumed here that there is a non-zero probability $(1-p-q)$ that after attempting to step, the random walker will not move. It is different from the simplest random walk considered above where each attempt was successful. So in this case the probability of forward and backward steps are not tightly coupled as above, and we have $p + q < 1$. Utilizing this recursion relation, one could also calculate the probability $P_N(m)$. But here we will use this approach for analyzing more realistic random walk systems that are closer to biological motors. So far we did not include time in our description of the random walk. Let us assume that each hopping for the random walker is taking place at average intervals $\Delta t = \tau$. The random walker makes N steps in the time $t = N\tau$. We can calculate the rates for jumping in the forward (right) and backward (left) directions at each attempt, and they are given by

$$u = p/\tau, \quad w = q/\tau. \tag{5.56}$$

The average position of the random walker changes with time. The Eq. (5.51) is still valid for the description of the average position for this random walk where not all attempts are successful, and we obtain that $< m >$ is linearly increasing with t,

$$\langle m \rangle = N\tau(u - w) = (u - w)t. \tag{5.57}$$

Then one can define a velocity of the random walker, $V \equiv d\langle m \rangle/dt$, which is equal to

$$V = u - w. \tag{5.58}$$

A convenient measure of randomness or stochasticity in the random walker motion is a *diffusion constant* which is defined as one half of the time derivative of the variance,

$$D \equiv \frac{1}{2}\frac{d(\langle m^2 \rangle - \langle m \rangle^2)}{dt}. \tag{5.59}$$

To calculate D let us consider a short time interval corresponding to the average time for one attempt for the random walker, $t = \tau$. Then we have

$$\langle m \rangle_1 = p - q = (u - w)\tau, \quad \langle m^2 \rangle_1 = (p + q) = (u + w)\tau, \tag{5.60}$$

where the subindex 1 is used here to underlie that these average quantities are calculated after one attempt. Then from Eq. (5.59) the diffusion constant is given by

$$D = \frac{u + w - (u - w)^2\tau}{2}. \tag{5.61}$$

The velocity V and the diffusion constant D are main dynamic parameters that characterize the random walk.

For biological motor proteins, time intervals between attempts are quite small, and we can modify the recursion relation (5.55) by assuming that τ is small and using the Taylor expansion. Then one derives the following expression for the probability of finding the random walker at the position m at time t, $P(m, t)$ (van Kampen 2001) [174],

$$\frac{dP(m, t)}{dt} = uP(m - 1, t) + wP(m + 1, t) - (u + w)P(m, t). \tag{5.62}$$

This is known as a continuous-time *master equation*, and it reflects the conservation of the probability at specific position m. The term master equation was given to this expression in 1940 because all properties of the system can be found from this relation (van Kampen 2001) [174]. This equation is very similar to chemical kinetic equations that we discussed above. Its physical meaning is that the temporal evolution of the probability function at the given site is determined by probability fluxes into this location and out of this location. One can see that the probability behaves similarly to concentrations of chemical molecules. One can find that for this continuous-time random walk, the dynamic properties are

$$V = u - w, \quad D = \frac{u + w}{2}. \tag{5.63}$$

These results agree with dynamic properties derived above for the discrete-time random walk in the limit of very small time intervals, $\tau \ll 1$.

The random walk ideas provide a powerful quantitative framework for analyzing mechanisms of motor proteins. The main advantage is that it allows us to connect microscopic transitions, including chemical reactions and mechanical displacements, of single molecular motors with their dynamic properties. We will discuss details of the application of the random walk concept for motor proteins in further chapters.

5.4 FIRST-PASSAGE PROCESSES

It is interesting to look in more detail into single-molecule experimental investigations of motor proteins as represented, e.g., by Fig. 3.10. One then realizes that in these experiments the motor protein molecules reside for some periods of time at specific locations and then jump to the next position. The motion looks random and it is called *stochastic*. The experiments measure quite precisely these residence times (time periods between jumps), which are also known as *dwell times*. But even when motors do not move they are involved in a series of chemical transitions. For example, these chemical reactions might include ATP binding, hydrolysis, and the release of hydrolysis products. It is important to note that dynamic properties, such as velocities and diffusion constants, are not measured directly but rather computed from these time periods and from the associated changes in the positions of motors. The distribution of dwell times contains full information on the mechanisms and dynamics of motor proteins. But how can we extract this microscopic information?

It seems natural that the language of random walks might be useful here. The question is how to connect molecular properties with the experimentally measured probability for the motor protein to reach a specific location along the cellular filament at time t for the first time. The critical words here are "for the first time." It was realized that this analysis can be done using the *first-passage processes*, which is a powerful tool for investigations of various processes in chemistry, physics, and biology (van Kampen 2001, Redner 2001) [174, 138]. The concept of first-passage processes also plays a crucial role for understanding biological molecular motors (Kolomeisky and Fisher 2007, Kolomeisky 2013) [84, 82].

To illustrate the application of first-passage ideas for motor proteins let us consider a simple model for the dynamics of single motors as presented in Fig. 5.7. The molecular motor is considered here as a random walker on the one-dimensional lattice segment consisting of $N + 1$ sites. Lattice sites $0 < i < N$ describe different chemical states of the motor protein when it is residing in a specific position along the filament. At initial time the random walker is found in the state i. The state N corresponds to the forward binding state, while the state 0 describes the backward binding site (see Fig. 5.7). Modern single-molecule experiments (Greenleaf et al. 2007, Veigel and Schmidt 2011) [63, 175] can measure quite precisely the arrival of the molecules to forward or backward binding positions. Our goal here is to show how the information on mechanisms of motor proteins can be obtained from distributions and probabilities of arrival events.

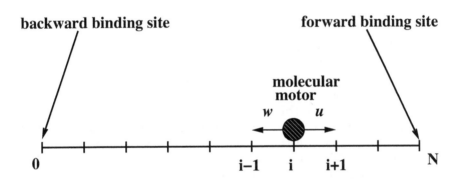

FIGURE 5.7 A simplified model for the application of first-passage processes for motor proteins. A molecular motor is viewed as a random walker that moves with the rate u in the forward direction and with the rate w backward. The site N corresponds to the forward binding position. The corresponding backward binding site is labeled 0.

We start our analysis of the model shown in Fig. 5.7 by introducing a new function $F_{N,i}(t)$, which is defined as a probability for the random walker to reach the site N for the first time at time t before reaching the site 0 if at $t = 0$ it started from the site i. The average time interval of the random walker jumping to the neighboring sites is equal to $\tau = 1/(u + w)$. Then for the probability distribution function $F_{N,i}(t)$ we can write

$$F_{N,i}(t + \tau) = \frac{u}{u + w} F_{N,i+1}(t) + \frac{w}{u + w} F_{N,i-1}(t). \tag{5.64}$$

The physical meaning of this equation is that in order to reach the forward binding site N the random walker should first forward to the site $i + 1$ with the probability $u/(u+w)$ or it has to hop backward to the site $i-1$, which can be accomplished with the probability $w/(u+w)$. Usually, the time interval is quite small and one can go to a continuous time limit, yielding

$$\frac{dF_{N,i}(t)}{dt} = uF_{N,i+1}(t) + wF_{N,i-1}(t) - (u+w)F_{N,i}(t). \qquad (5.65)$$

This expression is known as a *backward master equation*. It is interesting to note that although it is similar to the ordinary master equation (5.62) the backward master equation deviates significantly. It plays a central role in the first-passage analysis for any process.

In the Mathematical Appendix we show explicitly how to calculate the first-passage probability functions and how to apply them for getting dynamic properties of the random walker for the model given in Fig. 5.7. For the simple case of $w = 0$, when no backward transitions are allowed, we obtain an expression for the distribution of first-passage events if the starting position is at the site i,

$$F_{N,i}(t) = \frac{u^{N-i}t^{N-i-1}e^{-ut}}{(N-i-1)!}. \qquad (5.66)$$

Some of these dwell-time distribution functions are shown in Fig. 5.8. One can clearly see that they depend on the starting position. Simple exponential decay (solid curve) is observed if there is only one step before reaching the forward binding site ($i = 9$ and $N = 10$). For the starting position further away from the site N, the distribution functions are non-monotonic. The analysis of these distribution functions can provide direct information on the number of intermediate chemical states, which is very important for uncovering the mechanisms of biological molecular motors (Li and Kolomeisky 2013) [93].

First-passage distribution functions are also very useful for calculating dynamic properties of molecular motors. For example, we can define the overall probability of reaching the forward binding site as

$$\Pi_{N,i} = \int_0^\infty F_{N,i}(t)dt. \qquad (5.67)$$

This quantity is called a *splitting probability* (van Kampen 2001) [174]. It can be shown for general transition rates $u > w$ that (van Kampen 2001) [174]

$$\Pi_{N,i} = \frac{1 - (w/u)^i}{1 - (w/u)^N}. \qquad (5.68)$$

This is a very reasonable result. It suggests that the random walker that starts far away from the state N has a lower probability of hitting the forward binding site before reaching the site 0. But for $w = 0$ the probability is equal to one for any state, as expected since only forward motion is allowed. Using the first-passage probability functions we can also calculate the dwell time $\tau_{N,i}$ before the random walker will reach the site N. It is defined as

$$\tau_{N,i} = \frac{\int_0^\infty tF_{N,i}(t)dt}{\Pi_{N,i}}. \tag{5.69}$$

This quantity can be viewed as an average time before hitting the forward binding site (the numerator) under condition that it will be reached (the denominator). These times are also known as *mean first-passage times* (MFPT) (van Kampen 2001) [174]. It can be shown that this time is given by

$$\tau_{N,i} = \frac{1}{u-w}\left[i - N + \frac{2N}{1-(w/u)^N} - \frac{2i}{1-(w/u)^i}\right]. \tag{5.70}$$

For the situation with no backward steps ($w = 0$) the result is much simpler, $\tau_{N,i} = \frac{N-i}{u}$. In this case, the random walker steps forward and the average time for each jump is $1/u$, so that the total time is proportional to the number of steps between initial and final states.

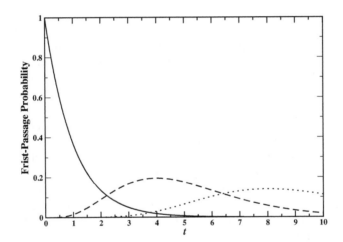

FIGURE 5.8 First-passage probability functions $F_{N,i}(t)$ for the random walk particle with $N = 10$ and with transition rates $u = 1$ and $w = 0$ for different starting positions. The random walker starts at the position i at $t = 0$ and it is found at the final state N at time t. The solid line corresponds to $i = 9$, the dashed lines is for $i = 5$, and the dotted curve is for $i = 1$.

This discussion shows that the first-passage concepts might be very productive for determining mechanisms of motor proteins. It allows us to fully analyze single-molecule experiments. The real biological motor systems are quite complex, but the same ideas can be applied for them. We discuss these issues in future chapters.

5.5 SUMMARY

In this chapter we discussed some theoretical methods that are needed for understanding the mechanisms of biological molecular motors. It was argued that since motor proteins operate under conditions that may deviate significantly from equilibrium, one has to employ non-equilibrium methods. In addition, we discussed how a dynamic description of motors can be obtained if a temporal behavior of motor proteins is available.

To start, we presented a brief review of the main methods of chemical kinetics. It was shown that the changes in concentrations of chemical species are directly related to rates of chemical processes. The explicit form of the temporal evolution of concentrations allows one to understand the mechanism and coupling of underlying chemical reactions. We argued that for motor protein systems, where a large number of chemical reactions are simultaneously taking place, one should be careful in the interpretation of experimental results since all processes are coupled. In addition, we discussed the dependence of chemical reaction rates on temperature, which is one of the most important approaches for getting microscopic information in complex systems with chemical processes.

Next, we analyzed the method of random walks. One can view the motion of motor proteins as hopping between different chemical and mechanical states that might be spatially separated. Then the ideas of random walks might be very useful because they provide a comprehensive quantitative description of biological motor dynamics. The concepts of the random walk were illustrated using simple examples.

Finally, the concept of first-passage processes was introduced. We argued that the nature of single-molecule experiments on motor proteins, where residence times and distributions of stepping events are measured with high precision, demand the application of this method. A simple model was presented, and we showed how to compute dynamic properties of molecular motors from distributions of dwell times at different states. This analysis directly connects microscopic properties of motor proteins, such as transition rates, with their dynamic characteristics.

5.6 MATHEMATICAL APPENDIX

5.6.1 *Irreversible Second-Order Chemical Reactions*

Let us consider a general form of the second-order chemical reaction as given by Eq. (5.10). We mostly follow here the method presented in (Houston 2001) [67]. The chemical rate law in the differential form can be written as

$$R = -\frac{d[A]}{dt} = k[A][B]. \tag{5.71}$$

It is assumed also that initially the concentrations of the reactants are equal to $[A](t = 0) = A_0$ and $[B](t = 0) = B_0$ with $B_0 \neq A_0$. We define a new function $x(t)$ as the number of A molecules that reacted at time t. Because of the stoichiometric relation in Eq. (5.10) we have

$$[A](t) = A_0 - x, \quad [B](t) = B_0 - x. \tag{5.72}$$

The rate law expression can then be written only in terms of the unknown function x,

$$\frac{dx}{dt} = k(A_0 - x)(B_0 - x). \tag{5.73}$$

This equation can be changed into the following,

$$\frac{dx}{(A_0 - x)(B_0 - x)} = kdt. \tag{5.74}$$

To simplify the further calculations one can use the following equality,

$$\frac{1}{(A_0 - x)(B_0 - x)} = \frac{1}{B_0 - A_0}\left[\frac{1}{A_0 - x} - \frac{1}{B_0 - x}\right]. \tag{5.75}$$

Then Eq. (5.75) can be easily integrated

$$\frac{1}{B_0 - A_0}\int_0^x \left[\frac{1}{A_0 - x} - \frac{1}{B_0 - x}\right] = \int_0^t kdt, \tag{5.76}$$

which leads to

$$\ln\left(\frac{A_0}{A_0 - x}\right) - \ln\left(\frac{B_0}{B_0 - x}\right) = (B_0 - A_0)kt. \tag{5.77}$$

Finally, using the definition of the function x from Eq. (5.73) we obtain

$$\ln\left(\frac{[B]A_0}{[A]B_0}\right) = (B_0 - A_0)kt. \tag{5.78}$$

In the limit of $A_0 \simeq B_0$ it can be shown that this expression reduces, as expected, to Eq. (5.14).

5.6.2 *Reversible Chemical Reactions*

For the simplest reversible chemical reaction, as described by Eq. (5.35), we can compute the temporal evolution of concentrations of A and B using the analysis similar to calculating properties of the second-order reactions (Houston 2001) [67]. The function $x(t)$, which gives the amount of A that reacted at time t, is again introduced. Then the concentrations of reactants and products are given by

$$[A](t) = A_0 - x, \quad [B](t) = B_0 + x. \tag{5.79}$$

There is also the equilibrium value of the function x, $x_e = x(t \to \infty)$. The equilibrium concentrations of A and B are related to this function via

$$A_e = A_0 - x_e, \quad B_e = B_0 + x_e. \tag{5.80}$$

The rate law Eq. (5.37) for this process can be rewritten as

$$\frac{dx}{dt} = k_1(A_0 - x) - k_{-1}(B_0 + x) = k_1(A_e + x_e - x) - k_{-1}(B_e - x_e + x), \quad (5.81)$$

which can be presented as follows:

$$\frac{dx}{dt} = (k_1 A_e - k_{-1} B_e) + k_1(x_e - x) + k_{-1}(x_e - x). \quad (5.82)$$

The first term on the right side of the equation is equal to zero because at equilibrium we have $k_1 A_e = k_{-1} B_e$. Then this expression simplifies into

$$\frac{dx}{dt} = -(k_1 + k_{-1})(x - x_e). \quad (5.83)$$

Now this equation can be easily integrated and we obtain

$$\ln\left(\frac{x_e - x}{x}\right) = -(k_1 + k_{-1})t, \quad (5.84)$$

which gives the explicit expression for the function x,

$$x(t) = x_e\left[1 - e^{-(k_1 + k_{-1})t}\right]. \quad (5.85)$$

Substituting this result into Eq. (5.79) leads to the final expressions for concentrations of A and B as given in Eqs. (5.41) and (5.42).

5.6.3 Calculations of Average Properties for the Simplest One-Dimensional Random Walk

To derive the average properties of the simplest one-dimensional random walk, shown in Fig. 5.4, we will use a mathematical result known as a *binomial theorem*,

$$(p + q)^N = \sum_{n=0}^{N} C_n^N p^n q^{N-n}, \quad (5.86)$$

where C_n^N is a binomial coefficient defined in Eq. (5.48). For this random walk model we have $p + q = 1$, and using Eq. (5.47) one might derive

$$\sum_{m=-N}^{N} P_N(m) = 1. \quad (5.87)$$

This is just an expected normalization result which confirms that the random walker, after N steps starting from the origin, with the probability one will be found on the lattice segment between sites $-N$ and N.

The calculation of the mean position of the random walker after N steps can be done if we recall Eq. (5.46). Let us first compute the average number of forward (right) steps $< n_r >$. The formal expression for this quantity is

$$\langle n_r \rangle = \sum_{n_r=0}^{N} n_r P_N(m) = \sum_{n_r=0}^{N} C_{n_r}^N n_r p^{n_r} q^{N-n_r}. \qquad (5.88)$$

To simplify calculations we can use the following mathematical trick,

$$n_r p^{n_r} = p \frac{\partial (p^{n_r})}{\partial p}. \qquad (5.89)$$

Then Eq. (5.88) can be written as

$$\langle n_r \rangle = p \frac{\partial}{\partial p} \left[\sum_{n_r=0}^{N} C_{n_r}^N p^{n_r} q^{N-n_r} \right]. \qquad (5.90)$$

The term in square brackets is the same as for the binomial theorem (see Eq. 5.86), so we obtain

$$\langle n_r \rangle = p \frac{\partial (p+q)^N}{\partial p} = pN(p+q)^{N-1} = pN. \qquad (5.91)$$

Similar arguments can be utilized to compute the average number of backward (left) steps, yielding

$$\langle n_l \rangle = Nq. \qquad (5.92)$$

Combining these results and Eq. (5.46) leads to the final formula for the average position of the random walker

$$\langle m \rangle = \langle n_r \rangle - \langle n_l \rangle = N(p-q) = N(2p-1), \qquad (5.93)$$

which is the same as Eq. (5.51).

We can calculate higher moments of the position of the random walker using similar arguments. For example, for the second moment ($\langle m^2 \rangle$) we can use $m = n_r - n_l = 2n_r - N$, which leads to

$$\langle m^2 \rangle = 4\langle n_r^2 \rangle + N^2 - 4N\langle n_r \rangle. \qquad (5.94)$$

We already calculated the average number of the forward steps, $< n_r >$, and now we need only to evaluate $< n_r^2 >$. By definition,

$$\langle n_r^2 \rangle = \sum_{n_r=0}^{N} n_r^2 P_N(m) = \sum_{n_r=0}^{N} C_{n_r}^N n_r^2 p^{n_r} q^{N-n_r}. \qquad (5.95)$$

Using the same mathematical trick with derivatives one can show that

$$n_r^2 p^{n_r} = n_r \left(p \frac{\partial}{\partial p} \right) (p^{n_r}) = \left(p \frac{\partial}{\partial p} \right)^2 (p^{n_r}). \qquad (5.96)$$

Substituting this result into Eq. (5.95) leads us to

$$\langle n_r^2 \rangle = \left(p\frac{\partial}{\partial p} \right)^2 \left[\sum_{n_r=0}^{N} C_{n_r}^N p^{n_r} q^{N-n_r} \right]. \tag{5.97}$$

With the help of the binomial theorem one can show that

$$\langle n_r^2 \rangle = \left(p\frac{\partial}{\partial p} \right)^2 (p+q)^N = \left(p\frac{\partial}{\partial p} \right) [Np(p+q)^{N-1}] = Np + N(N-1)p^2. \tag{5.98}$$

In a more convenient form this can be written as

$$\langle n_r^2 \rangle = (Np)^2 + Npq. \tag{5.99}$$

This expression can now be employed in Eq. (5.94) to obtain the final formula given in Eq. (5.52).

5.6.4 Calculations of First-Passage Probabilities and Dynamic Properties

There are several different approaches for calculating first-passage properties (van Kampen 2001, Redner 2001) [174, 138]. Here we show a method based on Laplace transformations. Our goal is to solve Eq. (5.65) for the model shown in Fig. 5.7. It is important also to take into account the boundary and initial conditions for this system, which are

$$
\begin{align}
F_{N,0}(t) &= 0, \text{ for all } t, \tag{5.100}\\
F_{N,N}(t) &= \delta(t), \tag{5.101}\\
F_{N,i}(t=0) &= 0, \text{ for } 1 \leq i \leq N-1. \tag{5.102}
\end{align}
$$

The physical meaning of the first condition is that if the random walker started at the site $i = 0$, its probability of reaching the right end site N before hitting the left end is zero by definition. The second condition implies that the particle starting at the site N reached its goal. The Dirac delta function is used here because of the normalization requirement that $\int_0^\infty F_{N,N}(t)dt = 1$. The third condition is simple to understand — for the random walker starting at any site $i \neq N$ at time zero the first-passage probability is zero.

For any first-passage probability function $F_{N,i}(t)$ we can define a Laplace transformation which creates a new function

$$\widetilde{F_{N,i}}(s) = \int_0^\infty e^{-st} F_{N,i}(t)dt. \tag{5.103}$$

The backward master equation (5.65) can be modified using Laplace transformations in the following way (omitting the variable s to simplify the notations),

$$(s+u+w)\widetilde{F_{N,i}} = u\widetilde{F_{N,i+1}} + w\widetilde{F_{N,i-1}}, \tag{5.104}$$

for $1 < i < N - 1$. At the same time, near the left end site we have

$$(s + u + w)\widetilde{F_{N,1}} = u\widetilde{F_{N,2}} \qquad (5.105)$$

because Eq. (5.100) implies that $\widetilde{F_{N,0}} = 0$. Near the right end site the expression is

$$(s + u + w)\widetilde{F_{N,N-1}} = u + w\widetilde{F_{N,N-2}}. \qquad (5.106)$$

This expression utilizes Eq. (5.101), which leads to $\widetilde{F_{N,N}} = 1$.

The advantage of using the Laplace transforms is that the original differential equations are substituted by algebraic equations which are much easier to solve. Here we will be looking for a solution in the form of

$$\widetilde{F_{N,i}} \simeq Ax^i, \qquad (5.107)$$

where parameters A and x should be determined from backward master equations as well as from boundary conditions. Substituting this ansatz into Eq. (5.104) leads to a quadratic equation with respect to the parameter x,

$$ux^2 - (s + u + w)x + w = 0. \qquad (5.108)$$

This has two roots:

$$x_1 = \frac{(s + u + w) + \sqrt{(s + u + w)^2 - 4uw}}{2u}, \qquad (5.109)$$

$$x_2 = \frac{(s + u + w) - \sqrt{(s + u + w)^2 - 4uw}}{2u}. \qquad (5.110)$$

It also suggests that the ansatz for the solution should be written as

$$\widetilde{F_{N,i}} = A_1 x_1^i + A_2 x_2^i. \qquad (5.111)$$

The unknown parameters A_1 and A_2 will be determined by substituting this ansatz into Eqs. (5.105) and (5.106), which produces,

$$(s + u + w)(A_1 x_1 + A_2 x_2) = u(A_1 x_1^2 + A_2 x_2 2), \qquad (5.112)$$
$$(s + u + w)(A_1 x_1^{N-1} + A_2 x_2^{N-1}) = u + w(A_1 x_1^{N-2} + A_2 x_2^{N-2}). \qquad (5.113)$$

This is a system of two equations with two unknowns, A_1 and A_2. The easiest way to solve it is to apply Eq. (5.109) in Eq. (5.113), which produces a simple relation $A_1 = -A_2$. Then using this relation and Eq. (5.109) in Eq. (5.114) yields

$$A_1 = -A_2 = \frac{1}{x_1^N - x_2^N}. \qquad (5.114)$$

Finally, we obtain an explicit formula for the Laplace transform of the first-passage probability functions,

$$\widetilde{F_{N,i}} = \frac{x_1^i - x_2^i}{x_1^N - x_2^N}. \qquad (5.115)$$

This can always be inverted (sometimes analytically, but always numerically) to get the original first-passage distribution functions. For example, let us consider the special case with $w = 0$, when the random walker can only make forward steps. In this case, $x_1 = (s + u)/u$ and $x_2 = 0$. Then we have

$$\widetilde{F_{N,i}} = \left(\frac{u}{s+u} \right)^{N-i},$$ (5.116)

which can easily be inverted: the result has been stated in Eq. (5.66).

Another advantage of utilizing Laplace transforms is that we can easily obtain analytical expressions for all dynamic properties, and there is no need to invert Laplace transforms. For example, the splitting probability can be found from

$$\Pi_{N,i} = \widetilde{F_{N,i}}(s = 0).$$ (5.117)

This allows us to easily obtain Eq. (5.68). The mean first-passage times in terms of Laplace transforms are given by

$$\tau_{N,i} = -\frac{1}{\Pi_{N,i}} \frac{d\widetilde{F_{N,i}}}{ds}(s = 0).$$ (5.118)

This expression was used in deriving the explicit result presented in Eq. (5.70).

CHAPTER 6

Motor Proteins as Enzymes

CONTENTS

6.1 INTRODUCTION

Motor proteins have two main biological functions. One is to develop mechanical forces for supporting transport of cellular species and for maintaining important biochemical processes associated with transfer of genetic information. We already discussed some fundamental features associated with exerting mechanical forces by biological molecular motors. The second function, which we did not mention yet, is to serve as enzymatic molecules. This means that motor proteins might speed up some specific chemical reactions in cells. Probably, the most important such reaction is the hydrolysis of ATP molecules or related compounds. These two functions of biological motors are tightly coupled with each other. The energy released in these catalyzed chemical processes is utilized by motors for doing the necessary mechanical work. So if we want to understand microscopic mechanisms of motor proteins, their catalytic properties are very important, and they should be discussed in more detail.

We would like to understand how the catalysis works from a fundamental point of view and why it is relevant for a motor protein's dynamics. More specifically, the following questions regarding the enzymatic activity of biological molecular motors need to be answered:

1. What is the catalysis and why can catalytic molecules accelerate chemical reactions without being consumed or produced?

2. What is so special about the biological catalysts that are called enzymes?

3. How do we quantitatively describe the dynamics of enzymatic molecules?

4. What is the role of enzyme catalysis for motor proteins?

We concentrate on more fundamental features of the catalysis, and we will be more quantitative in our efforts to describe dynamics of enzymatic systems.

6.2   CATALYSIS

Catalysis is a set of unique physical-chemical phenomena when special compounds, which are called *catalysts*, modify the rates of particular chemical reactions without being consumed or created (Somorjai and Li 2010) [150]. Catalytic processes have been known to humans from ancient times. The production of alcohol from sugar is the first and still very significant example. Catalysis is so critically important that our modern life cannot be imagined without use of catalysts in all branches of industry, including food production, medicine, ecology, and materials production. Very different substances might be catalysts, ranging from metals to acid or base solutions. Probably, the most famous example of catalysts from our everyday life are catalytic converters in our cars that decrease the amount of toxic exhaust gases by accelerating reactions of oxidation.

The term *catalysis* was introduced in 1835 by the Swedish scientist Jons Jacob Berzelius (see Fig. 6.1), and it comes from Greek words that mean "dissolution" or "decomposition." Berzelius is one of the most famous scientists in the 19th century because he is one of the founders of modern chemistry. One of his most notable contributions to science was the development of chemical notations for formulas as we use them now. In early studies of catalysis, scientists thought that the catalytic processes were controlled mostly by physical forces like heat or electric fields. But in 1833 French scientists Anselme Payen and Jean-Francois Persoz discovered that the acceleration of a chemical reaction that transformed starch into a mixture of sugar molecules was due to the action of a special substance which is known now as *amylase* (Payen and Persoz 1833) [123]. It was the first isolated and investigated enzyme molecule. The discovery of catalysts have shown the importance of chemical interactions in catalytic processes. It is now widely accepted that both physical and chemical interactions are equally important for catalytic processes.

Catalysis has been widely investigated, both experimentally and theoretically, and although the full microscopic picture of this phenomenon is still not complete (Somorjai and Li 2010) [150], the current view of its main mechanism is the following. As we discussed in the previous chapter, the rate of a chemical reaction is determined by the height of the barrier along the reaction coordinate; see Fig. 6.2. What is important in catalytic processes is that the free energies of the reactants and products are not changed. However, the

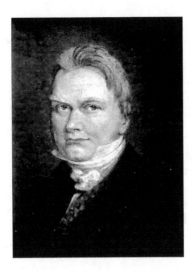

FIGURE 6.1 The famous Swedish chemist Jons Jacob Berzelius (1779–1848) who was one of the pioneers in studies of catalytic phenomena in the 19th century.

catalyst opens a new free-energy pathway for the reaction, one with lower barriers, as shown in Fig. 6.2. This leads to an increase in the rate of formation of products. The main idea of catalysis is similar to a problem that hiking tourists face in mountain regions. It is frequently faster and easier to bypass the mountain instead of trying to go over it directly. In reality, the free-energy picture of catalysis obviously is significantly more complicated than the simple scheme presented in Fig. 6.2. It involves a complex mixture of various physical and chemical interactions. Typical catalytic processes might also include many transitions and intermediate states. This is true for all enzymatic processes and especially for motor proteins.

Analyzing the free-energy picture of catalytic processes, as given in Fig. 6.2, two important observations can be made. First, because the free-energy difference between the products and reactants do not change in catalytic processes, one might conclude that the catalyst accelerates *both* forward and backward chemical processes (Somorjai and Li 2010, Houston 2001) [150, 67]. Due to the *principle of microscopic reversibility* the backward chemical reaction must always follow the same pathway as the forward process. This is a result of the fact that fundamental equations that govern chemical and physical systems are fully time reversible, i.e., the main properties of systems do not change if the sign of the time changes. For motor proteins, this means that they might accelerate both the hydrolysis of ATP as well as the synthesis of ATP molecules from ADP and inorganic phosphate. This has been experimentally observed in F_0F_1 ATP synthase rotary motors (Itoh et al. 2004,

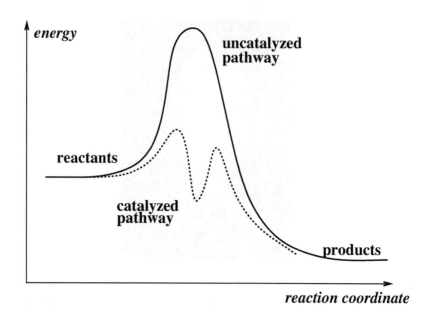

FIGURE 6.2 A schematic view of the effect of catalysis on chemical reactions. The solid line represents the free-energy pathway for the uncatalyzed process, while the dashed line shows the catalytic pathway with an intermediate state for the identical overall reaction.

Rondelez et al. 2005) [74, 135]. In addition, similar observations were made for some kinesin motor proteins (Cochran et al. 2005, Hackney 2005) [32, 64]. It is important to note that in many situations the backward reaction, even accelerated by the catalysis, is still too slow to be observed on experimental time scales. Probably, this is the case for the majority of motor protein systems in live cells. However, the reversibility of chemical reactions that are catalyzed by molecular motors cannot be neglected since it might lead to serious errors in understanding their mechanisms (Kolomeisky and Fisher 2007, Kolomeisky 2013) [84, 82].

The second important conclusion from the free-energy description of catalytic processes is that catalysis *does not always* lead to faster chemical reactions. On the contrary, there are substances that might significantly slow down chemical reactions (Somorjai and Li 2010, Houston 2001, Tinoco et al. 2003) [150, 67, 164]. They are generally called *inhibitors*. There are many possible mechanisms of how inhibitors might decrease rates of specific chemical reactions. For example, inhibitors might bind to catalysts and block their activities. We can also understand another possible method of inhibiting the chemical reaction by using the simple scheme in Fig. 6.2. The inhibitor might lead to a very stable intermediate state which serves as a local trap so that the reaction does not proceed at all. Inhibition is important for various biological and industrial processes. Many food additives, e.g., acids such as vinegar and lemon juice, are catalytic inhibitors that slow down the undesired processes that lead to food spoiling.

6.3 ENZYMATIC PROCESSES

Enzymes are biological catalysts that have an outstanding ability to accelerate biologically important chemical reactions (Cornish-Bowden 2012) [34]. To illustrate this superior effectiveness of biological catalysts let us consider the following example (Tinoco et al. 2003) [164]. Hydrogen peroxide at room temperature decomposes into water and oxygen molecules via the reaction

$$2H_2O_2 \rightleftharpoons 2H_2O + O_2. \tag{6.1}$$

This reaction is very slow. One can go to a pharmacy to buy an aqueous solution of hydrogen peroxide, the well-known antimicrobial agent, which can stay active for long periods of time. But if we add few drops of bromide solution to the hydrogen peroxide system, the reaction will go 10,000 times faster because Br^- is a catalyst for this reaction. However, adding the enzyme catalase speeds up the reaction by 15 orders of magnitude! This is one of the fastest enzymatic processes. It clearly shows how effective biological catalysts are.

To understand why enzymes are such remarkable catalysts we recall that most of them are protein molecules that have complex biological structures. It is known that the reaction takes place in a special region of the enzyme which is known as the *active site*. The structure of the active site is such that it allows efficient binding of the reactants, which are called *substrates*, and the further process of creating and removing product molecules (Cornish-Bowden 2012) [34]. It has been argued that this fit between structures of active sites of enzymes and structures of substrates is the main reason for extremely high efficiency of biological catalytic processes. This idea is known as a "lock-and-key" concept for enzymatic activity (Cornish–Bowden 2012) [34]. Because enzymes are such powerful catalysts, very low concentrations of active protein molecules are frequently needed, which is a great advantage for cells. As a result, in many cases there are only few copies of enzyme molecules per cell. This is extremely useful for biological systems since a large variety of different enzymes can function simultaneously in the cell, supporting all necessary processes and without interfering with each other.

The remarkable efficiency and specificity of enzyme molecules is reflected in their dynamics. Experiments show that most enzymes have universal chemical kinetic properties. The main properties of enzymatic kinetics were uncovered in 1913 by the German scientist Leonor Michaelis (Fig. 6.3) and the Canadian biochemist Maud Menten (Fig. 6.4) (Michaelis and Menten 1913) [112]. There are several interesting facts about both of them. Michaelis found that thioglycolic acid might be used for dissolving keratin, which is the main protein in hair. It was the beginning of a revolution in the hair-related cosmetics industry. Maud Menten was one of the first Canadian women who obtained a medical degree. But during her times, women were not allowed to do research in Canada, so she worked most of her life in the United States. But the famous work was done by Michaelis and Menten when they worked together in Germany. The theoretical analysis of Michaelis and Menten was later further extended by British scientists G.E. Briggs and J.B.S. Haldane (Briggs and Haldane 1925) [24]. It is now called a *Michaelis–Menten mechanism*, and it is the most important fundamental part of modern enzymatic kinetics (Cornish–Bowden 2012) [34].

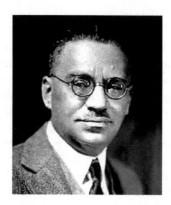

FIGURE 6.3   The German biochemist and biophysicist Leonor Michaelis (1875–1949) who developed the foundations of enzymatic kinetics. He is responsible for the Michaelis–Menten mechanism.

Michaelis and Menten were investigating the process of conversion of one type of sugar molecules, sucrose, into a mixture of two other sugars, glucose and fructose, catalyzed by the yeast enzyme invertase. They noticed that the rate of reaction at low concentrations of the substrate, $[S] \ll 1$, was proportional to the amount of the enzyme, $[E]$. In addition, at the same conditions of low substrate concentration for a fixed concentration of enzyme, they found that the reaction rate was linear with $[S]$. Furthermore, at higher concentrations of the substrate the reaction rate reached a plateau. Similar observations were made for many other enzyme-catalyzed chemical reactions. In Fig. 3.1B the reaction rate of ATP hydrolysis catalyzed by the kinesin-related Ncd motor protein shows the same behavior as found by Michaelis and Menten for the yeast enzyme invertase. In this case, ATP plays the role of the substrate and ADP is the monitored product of the chemical reaction (Foster and Gilbert 2000) [56].

To explain these observations, Michaelis and Menten proposed the follow-

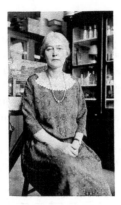

FIGURE 6.4 The famous Canadian biochemist Maud Menten (1879–1960), who together with L. Michaelis, developed the foundations of enzymatic kinetics.

ing simple kinetic scheme (Houston 2001) [67],

$$E + S \underset{k_{-1}}{\overset{k_1}{\rightleftharpoons}} ES, \tag{6.2}$$

$$ES \overset{k_2}{\rightarrow} P + E. \tag{6.3}$$

Note that the second reaction is supposed to be effectively irreversible so that k_2 can be neglected. Here E, S, ES, and P specify enzyme, substrate, enzyme–substrate complex, and product molecules, respectively. This mechanism implies that the enzyme can reversibly bind to the substrate, producing the enzyme–substrate complex. From this complex the enzyme might convert the substrate into the final product state. Chemical kinetic equations for this scheme can be analyzed using the steady-state approximation that we discussed in the previous chapter. It can be shown (see Mathematical Appendix for details) that the initial rate of the reaction, when the amount of product is still small, can be written as

$$R_0 = \left[\frac{d[\text{P}]}{dt}\right]_{t \to 0} = \frac{V_{max}}{1 + K_M/S_0}. \tag{6.4}$$

It is known as the *Michaelis–Menten equation*. In this expression,

$$V_{max} = k_2 E_0, \tag{6.5}$$

and

$$K_M = \frac{k_{-1} + k_2}{k_1}. \tag{6.6}$$

Also, E_0 and S_0 are the initial concentrations of the enzyme and substrate, respectively, while V_{max} is the maximal rate of the reaction which can be achieved for very large initial amounts of the substrate, $S_0 \gg 1$. The second stage of the process in Eq. (6.3) is a rate-limiting step of the whole reaction for this set of conditions. For low initial concentrations of the substrate, the first step becomes rate limiting, $R_0 \simeq k_1 E_0 S_0$, since the reaction rate k_2, which is sometimes called a *turnover number*, is usually quite large (Houston 2001) [67]. This agrees with the experimental observations presented above. The parameter K_M is known as the *Michaelis constant*, and it has the physical meaning of a concentration of the substrate at which the reaction rate is equal to one half of the maximal rate, $R_0 = V_{max}/2$. For practical analysis of experimental data, the Michaelis–Menten equation is frequently written in the linearized form,

$$\frac{1}{R_0} = \frac{1}{V_{max}} + \frac{K_M}{V_{max} S_0}, \tag{6.7}$$

which is called a *Lineweaver–Burk equation*.

The Michaelis–Menten approach is convenient also for analyzing more complex processes associated with enzymatic kinetics such as inhibition when the overall reaction rate might slow down (Houston 2001, Tinoco et al. 2003) [67, 164]. There are many possible inhibition mechanisms, but usually two specific cases are considered. The first one is called a *competitive inhibition*, and the kinetic scheme for this process is

$$\text{E} + \text{S} \; \underset{k_{-1}}{\overset{k_1}{\rightleftharpoons}} \; \text{ES}, \tag{6.8}$$

$$\text{ES} \; \overset{k_2}{\rightarrow} \; \text{P} + \text{E}. \tag{6.9}$$

$$\text{E} + \text{I} \; \underset{k_{-3}}{\overset{k_3}{\rightleftharpoons}} \; \text{EI}. \tag{6.10}$$

It is assumed that in this process a compound I, which is called an inhibitor, might react with the enzyme to quickly establish equilibrium. The enzyme in the complex EI cannot catalyze the reaction because the inhibitor binds to the active site of the catalyst. Then the initial rate of the reaction, as derived in the Mathematical Appendix, is equal to

$$R_0 = \left[\frac{d[P]}{dt}\right]_{t \to 0} = \frac{V_{max}}{1 + (K_M/S_0)\,(1 + [I]K_I)}, \tag{6.11}$$

where

$$K_I = \frac{k_3}{k_{-3}} = \frac{[EI]}{[E][I]}, \tag{6.12}$$

is the equilibrium constant for the inhibitor binding to enzyme molecules. The effect of inhibition is shown in Fig. 6.5. The competitive inhibition does not affect the maximal reaction rate, but it requires more substrate to compensate for enzyme molecules that do not function due to binding to the inhibitor.

The second inhibition mechanism is called a *non-competitive mechanism*

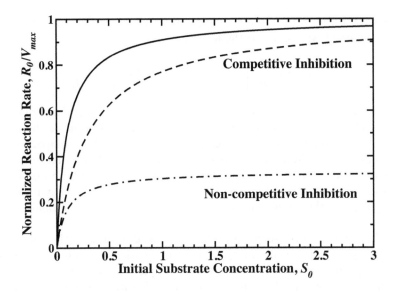

FIGURE 6.5 Michaelis–Menten analysis of various enzymatic processes. Normalized reaction rates as a function of the initial concentration of the substrate molecules are shown for a simple Michaelis–Menten mechanism utilizing Eq. (6.4) [solid curve], utilizing Eq. (6.11) for the competitive inhibition [dashed curve], and utilizing Eq. (6.18) for the non-competitive inhibition [dash-dotted curve]. The parameters used for calculations are $K_M = 0.1$, $[I] = 1$ and $K_I = 2$ in arbitrary units.

because the inhibitor does not bind the enzyme molecule at the active site but rather in another position. The kinetic scheme for this mechanism is

$$E + S \overset{k_1}{\underset{k_{-1}}{\rightleftharpoons}} ES, \tag{6.13}$$

$$ES \overset{k_2}{\rightarrow} P + E, \tag{6.14}$$

$$E + I \overset{k_3}{\underset{k_{-3}}{\rightleftharpoons}} EI, \tag{6.15}$$

$$ES + I \overset{k_4}{\underset{k_{-4}}{\rightleftharpoons}} ESI. \tag{6.16}$$

In this case, the inhibitor might also attach to the enzyme–substrate complex, and it is reasonable to assume that the equilibrium constants for the last two reactions are the same,

$$K_I = \frac{k_3}{k_{-3}} = \frac{[EI]}{[E][I]} = \frac{k_4}{k_{-4}} = \frac{[ESI]}{[ES][I]}. \tag{6.17}$$

Then the initial rate of the enzymatic reaction is modified, as shown in the Mathematical Appendix, in the following way

$$R_0 = \left[\frac{d[P]}{dt}\right]_{t\to 0} = \frac{V_{max}}{[1 + (K_M/S_0)]\,[1 + [I]K_I]}. \tag{6.18}$$

The expression for V_{max} is the same as before, but the maximal rate for this process is smaller by the factor $1 + [I]K_I$ as can be seen in the limit of very large initial concentrations of the substrate, $S_0 \gg 1$. The comparison of two mechanisms of inhibition, as presented in Fig. 6.5, shows that the maximal rate of the reaction decreases for the non-competitive inhibition process. The main reason for this is the lowering of the amount of the enzyme–substrate complex, i.e., the active form of the enzyme, from which the final product is made.

One of the most surprising observations is that the Michaelis–Menten mechanism works for almost all known enzymatically catalyzed reactions. It is the approximate description of a very simple kinetic scheme, while real biological processes involve complex networks of states (Cornish–Bowden 2012) [34]. It can be argued (Kolomeisky 2011) [81], that the behavior of any general enzymatic system should be quite similar to the Michaelis–Menten dynamics. If the concentration of the substrate is very low, then the reaction of substrate binding is always rate-limiting, and the linear dependence on S_0 is expected, independently of the complexity of enzymatic network. For large concentrations of the substrate, other processes become more important, leading to the reaction rate saturation as a function of S_0. As a result, the dependence of R_0 on the substrate concentration should generally look very similarly to the hyperbolic function predicted by Michaelis and Menten. One should also mention that the Michaelis–Menten relations can be obtained from a single-molecule perspective (see the Mathematical Appendix). This is very important for motor proteins because a large amount of information on their mechanisms comes from analysis of single-molecule experiments (Kolomeisky 2013) [82].

This brief analysis suggests that enzymatic processes are very important for motor proteins. It allows biological molecular motors not only to obtain the necessary chemical energy, but also to get it very quickly so that their functions can be efficiently supported. One can also see that the dynamic features and efficiency of motor proteins can be easily tuned by modifying their enzymatic properties.

6.4 SUMMARY

In this chapter we discussed the foundations of catalysis and the application of these ideas and concepts to enzymatic processes. Catalysis is a complex physical-chemical process which allows significant speedup of the chemical reactions. We argued that catalysts do not change free energies of the reactants and products but rather provide new pathways between initial and final states along which the reaction might proceed much faster. This has important consequences including the fact that catalysis affects forward and backward processes equally, and some reactions might even slow down the rate of product formation.

Next, we discussed in more detail enzymes (or biological catalysts) which are much more efficient and selective in their functions. The reason for this is the complex structure of protein molecules that allows catalytic processes to take place in specific locations known as active sites. The highly efficient nature of enzyme molecules also leads to specific dynamic properties that may be well described by the Michaelis–Menten mechanism. We analyzed carefully the origin of the Michaelis–Menten mechanism and its applications to more realistic enzymatic properties. It was shown also that the Michaelis–Menten equation is correct even at the single-molecule level. Finally, it was argued that it is very important for motor proteins to also be enzymes since the energy of catalyzed reactions might be accessible for biological molecular motors on very short time scales.

6.5 MATHEMATICAL APPENDIX

6.5.1 *Michaelis–Menten Mechanism*

The Michaelis–Menten approach is based on chemical kinetic analysis of the scheme presented in Eqs. (6.2) and (6.3):

$$\text{E} + \text{S} \underset{k_{-1}}{\overset{k_1}{\rightleftharpoons}} \text{ES}, \tag{6.19}$$

$$\text{ES} \overset{k_2}{\rightarrow} \text{P} + \text{E}. \tag{6.20}$$

For the enzyme–substrate complex we can write,

$$\frac{d[ES]}{dt} = k_1[E][S] - (k_{-1} + k_2)[ES], \tag{6.21}$$

while the rate of creating the product is given by

$$\frac{d[P]}{dt} = k_2[ES]. \tag{6.22}$$

Now we can use the steady-state approximation (SSA) that was discussed in Chapter 5. According to SSA, the rate of change for the intermediate compound, ES in this case, is assumed to be equal to zero. It leads to

$$\frac{d[ES]}{dt} = 0 = k_1[E][S] - (k_{-1} + k_2)[ES]. \tag{6.23}$$

The chemical process started with initial concentrations of enzyme and substrate as E_0 and S_0, respectively. The material balance conditions require that

$$E_0 = [E] + [ES], \tag{6.24}$$

and

$$S_0 = [S] + [ES] + [P]. \tag{6.25}$$

For enzymatic reactions the amount of the catalysts is always much smaller than the amount of the substrate, or $E_0 \ll S_0$. Obviously, the concentration of the intermediate complex ES is even smaller, $[ES] < E_0$. In addition, we are interested in the reaction rate at early times when almost no product molecules are created, $[P] \simeq 0$. Taking this into account and substituting Eqs. (6.24) and (6.25) into Eq. (6.23) we derive,

$$[ES] \simeq \frac{k_1 E_0 S_0}{k_1 S_0 + k_{-1} + k_2}. \tag{6.26}$$

Then using Eq. (6.20) the final expression for the rate of the enzymatic process at $t \to 0$, as given in Eq. (6.4), is obtained.

6.5.2 Inhibition Processes

Here we extend the Michaelis–Menten analysis to account for possible inhibition processes. First, we start with the competitive inhibition as described by Eqs. (6.8)–(6.10). The change in the concentration of the enzyme–inhibitor complex EI is given by

$$\frac{d[EI]}{dt} = k_3[E][I] - k_{-3}[EI]. \tag{6.27}$$

We can again apply the SSA method, and in this system two compounds, ES and EI, can be treated as intermediate. From the stationary condition, $d[EI]/dt = 0$, it can be shown that

$$[EI] = K_I[I][E], \tag{6.28}$$

where the equilibrium constant K_I is given in Eq. (6.12). The material balance condition for this system is modified as

$$E_0 = [E] + [ES] + [EI] = [E](1 + K_I[I]) + [ES]. \tag{6.29}$$

It can be shown that

$$[E] = \frac{E_0 - [ES]}{(1 + K_I[I])}. \tag{6.30}$$

Employing this result in the SSA expression for ES [see Eq. (6.23)] we derive

$$[ES] \simeq \frac{k_1 E_0 S_0}{k_1 S_0 + (k_{-1} + k_2)(1 + K_I[I])}. \tag{6.31}$$

Finally, substituting this expression into Eq. (6.20) yields the initial chemical rate for the competitive inhibition as given in Eq. (6.11).

For the non-competitive inhibition, as specified by chemical reactions in

Eqs. (6.13)–(6.16), the analysis is very similar. The rate of creation of the ESI complex is

$$\frac{d[ESI]}{dt} = k_4[ES][I] - k_{-4}[ESI].$$ (6.32)

The SSA method is then utilized, and ES, EI, and ESI are considered to be the intermediate substances which quickly reach the steady-state conditions. The assumption specified in Eq. (6.17) and the stationary condition for ESI leads us to

$$[ESI] = K_I[I][ES].$$ (6.33)

The material balance for enzyme species for this system is different,

$$E_0 = [E] + [ES] + [EI] + [ESI].$$ (6.34)

Using Eqs. (6.26) and (6.31) we obtain

$$E_0 = (1 + K_I[I])([E] + [ES]),$$ (6.35)

which yields

$$[E] = \frac{E_0}{(1 + K_I[I])} - [ES].$$ (6.36)

Substituting this expression into Eq. (6.23) gives us

$$[ES] \simeq \frac{k_1 E_0 S_0}{(k_1 S_0 + k_{-1} + k_2)(1 + K_I[I])}.$$ (6.37)

Utilizing this result in Eq. (6.20) leads to the final formula for the initial chemical rate in the system with non-competitive inhibition as presented by Eq. (6.18).

6.5.3 *Single-Molecule Derivation of the Michaelis–Menten Equation*

Let us a consider a single enzyme molecule in the solution with the initial concentration $[S] = S_0$ of the substrate molecules. For example, the enzyme could be the kinesin motor protein and the substrate would correspond to the ATP. The enzyme molecule can reversibly bind to the substrate, and it might lead to synthesis of the product. We can distinguish three possible states for the system as described by the following scheme,

$$0 \underset{w_1}{\overset{u_1}{\rightleftharpoons}} 1 \overset{u_2}{\rightarrow} 2.$$ (6.38)

The state 0 corresponds to the free enzyme, the state 1 describes the bound enzyme, and the state 2 is almost identical to the state 0 (enzyme is not bound) but with the only difference that there is one more product molecule P in this state in comparison with the state 0. The transition rate from the state 0 to the state 1 is equal to u_1, the reversed process has the rate w_1, and the rate to go from the state 1 to the state 2 is given by u_2.

We are interested in the average time it takes for the system to go from the state 0 to the state 2. As we discussed in Chapter 5, this quantity corresponds to the first-passage time. One can introduce a function $F_i(t)$ as the probability for the system to reach the state 2 if at time $t = 0$ the system was in the state i $(i = 0, 1, 2)$. These functions are governed by the *backward master equations*:

$$\frac{dF_0(t)}{dt} = u_1 F_1(t) - u_1 F_0(t),$$

$$\frac{dF_1(t)}{dt} = w_1 F_0(t) + u_2 F_2(t) - (u_2 + w_1) F_1(t). \tag{6.39}$$

In addition, we have the following boundary condition, $F_2(t) = \delta(t)$. The physical meaning of this condition is that if we start the process from the state 2 our goal is accomplished already at $t = 0$. These equations can be solved by employing the Laplace transformation method, as discussed in the previous chapter. We define

$$\widetilde{F_i}(s) = \int_0^\infty e^{-st} F_i(t) dt, \tag{6.40}$$

for $i = 0, 1, 2$. One can see immediately that $\widetilde{F_2}(s) = 1$. Then master equations can be written in the simpler form,

$$(s + u_1)\widetilde{F_0} = u_1 \widetilde{F_1},$$

$$(s + u_2 + w_1)\widetilde{F_1} = w_1 \widetilde{F_0} + u_2. \tag{6.41}$$

This system of algebraic equations can be easily solved yielding

$$\widetilde{F_0}(s) = \frac{u_1 u_2}{s^2 + s(u_1 + u_2 + w_1) + u_1 u_2}. \tag{6.42}$$

The mean first-passage time τ_0 to reach the state 2 from the state 0 is given by

$$\tau_0 = -\left[\frac{d\widetilde{F_0}(s)}{ds}\right]_{s=0}. \tag{6.43}$$

From Eq. (6.40) we obtain

$$\tau_0 = \frac{u_1 + u_2 + w_1}{u_1 u_2}. \tag{6.44}$$

The physical meaning of this time is that it represents the average time of the enzymatic cycle for the chemical reaction of making molecules P. The inverse of this quantity is the reaction rate per one enzymatic molecule,

$$r_0 = 1/\tau_0. \tag{6.45}$$

The macroscopic chemical rate is obtained by multiplying the molecular rate by the concentration of enzyme molecules,

$$R_0 = r_0[E]. \tag{6.46}$$

Finally, we should connect transition rates u_1, u_2, and w_1 with the rate constants utilized in the Michaelis–Menten analysis,

$$u_1 = k_1[S], \quad u_2 = k_2, \quad w_1 = k_{-1}. \tag{6.47}$$

Note that here we are using the single-molecule view of the process from the perspective of the enzyme molecule. For this reason, the first rate must be proportional to the amount of the substrate molecules. Finally, assembling together Eqs. (6.42)–(6.45) we can easily obtain the Michaelis–Menten equation for the initial chemical reaction rate as given in Eq. (6.4).

CHAPTER 7

Theory for Motor Proteins: Continuum Ratchets

CONTENTS

7.1 INTRODUCTION

As we already discussed in Chapter 3, motor proteins have been intensively investigated by a variety of different methods and techniques (Howard 2001, Greenleaf et al. 2007, Veigel and Schmidt 2011, Kolomeisky and Fisher 2007, Kolomeisky 2013, Chowdhury 2013) [68, 63, 175, 84, 82, 30]. The quantity of collected experimental information on biological molecular motors is quite large, but it is not well rationalized. These observations stimulated multiple attempts to develop microscopic understanding of processes that govern the functioning of motor proteins. Several theoretical ideas have been proposed and analyzed (Howard 2001, Kolomeisky and Fisher 2007, Kolomeisky 2013, Chowdhury 2013, Julicher et al. 1997) [68, 84, 82, 30, 76]. It is important to note that many aspects of motor proteins' activities are known with quite a high degree of precision. So it should definitely help us in testing various theoretical proposals. In addition, the fundamental concepts from physics and chemistry discussed in previous chapters should assist us in evaluation of the feasibility of different theoretical ideas concerning motor proteins. In this chapter, as well as in the next, we critically discuss major theoretical approaches that have been employed for describing dynamics and properties of biological molecular motors.

The main goal of all theoretical models of motor proteins is to provide a quantitative link between biochemical processes associated with molecular motors and their mechanical and dynamic properties. Crucial questions are: If we know the rates of the chemical reactions in which motor proteins participate, and the concentrations of all relevant species in the system, can we predict their velocities, diffusion constants, forces, and enzymatic efficiencies? How much energy is needed to sustain the dynamics of molecular motors observed in biological cells? How do different motors interact with each other and what are the main principles governing the collective properties of motor proteins? Clarifying all these issues will provide a better microscopic understanding of the mechanisms of energy conversion in biological molecular motors.

In developing theoretical models for motor proteins, one should remember that they must obey strict fundamental requirements. Only well-founded ideas can be utilized for understanding these complex phenomena. This is the main reason why we discussed in detail fundamental physical-chemical concepts before proceeding to the analysis of specific theoretical methods for biological molecular motors. We already outlined conditions for theoretical models in Chapter 1, so here we just recall that a successful theoretical framework must properly take into account various symmetries of the motor protein systems. They include periodicity and polarity of molecular tracks—microtubules, actin filaments, and nucleic acids in most cases can be viewed as polar, periodic structures with chemically different tail and head regions. A successful theoretical approach should provide a *quantitative* description of all properties of motor proteins, and it should also be able to make experimentally testable quantitative predictions. Probably, the most important feature of successful theories for motor proteins is that they should not violate basic laws of physics and chemistry. As an example, one cannot use the equilibrium model to describe biological molecular motors which function at strongly non-equilibrium conditions. One also cannot assume that chemical reactions associated with motor proteins are irreversible since chemical processes generally proceed in both directions.

To continue to develop theoretical ideas, we note that most experimentally studied motor proteins typically function in cells in a linear fashion. They move consistently along cytoskeleton protein filaments (microtubules or actin filaments), and along the nucleic acids (DNA or RNA). These biological tracks are polymers so that the dynamics of biological molecular motors can be viewed as effective one-dimensional motion. This is a significant simplification for the complex problem of quantitative description of motor proteins. All present theoretical approaches for molecular motors have adopted this point of view, although the implementations of this picture vary significantly (Howard 2001, Kolomeisky and Fisher 2007, Kolomeisky 2013, Julicher et al. 1997, Chowdhury 2013) [68, 84, 82, 76, 30].

There are two main ideas on how motor proteins function. One of them postulates that the molecular motor proceeds in a time-dependent one-dimensional free-energy landscape created by multiple chemical processes and various physical interactions in the system. The free-energy landscape is time-dependent because the motor's motion along one continuum potential surface can be interrupted by a chemical reaction that might switch the motor protein to another potential surface (Julicher et al. 1997, Howard 2001, Kolomeisky and Fisher 2007, Kolomeisky 2013, Chowdhury 2013) [76, 68, 84, 82, 30]. This method we call a *continuum ratchet approach*, and it will be discussed in detail in this chapter.

A different theoretical approach suggests that the motion of motor proteins can be described by networks of spatially varying specific biochemical states connected by discrete stochastic transitions (Kolomeisky and Fisher 2007, Kolomeisky 2013, Chowdhury 2013) [84, 82, 30]. This *discrete-state stochastic approach* will be fully analyzed in the next chapter.

7.2 CONTINUUM RATCHET POTENTIALS

The theoretical method of continuum ratchet potentials, also known as *thermal ratchet models* or *Markov–Fokker–Planck models*, has its origin in the work of famous Austrian scientist of Polish origin Marian von Smoluchowski (see Fig. 7.1). In the early years of the 20th century he developed the first theoretical description of random motion of molecules in liquids or gases, which is known as Brownian motion (Smoluchowski 1906) [149]. Similar ideas were independently proposed by Albert Einstein at approximately the same time (Einstein 1905) [48]. Despite Smoluchowski's short scientific career (he died in 1917 at the age of 45 from dysentery), Smoluchowski is considered to be one of the most influential scientists in modern physics and chemistry. He is the founder of the modern kinetic theory of matter, he developed fundamental concepts in chemical kinetics and diffusion, and he was also one of the first who applied the method of stochastic processes for various phenomena in physics, chemistry and biology.

Another inspiration for continuum description of motor proteins came from the concept of "thermal ratchet" as developed by the American physicist Richard Feynman (Fig. 7.2) in his lectures (Feynman et al. 1966) [52]. Feynman is one of the best-known theoretical physicists in the 20th century. He received a Nobel Prize in Physics in 1965 for fundamental contributions in quantum electrodynamics, but he also made significant contributions in many other areas of physics.

The main idea of thermal ratchet models is to view the biological molecular motor as a particle that travels along several spatially parallel free-energy potential surfaces, as shown in Fig. 7.3. Probably, one of the first implementations of this idea was made in 1987 (Chen 1987) [29]. These continuum potentials are periodic and generally asymmetric. This is due to the fact that these are effective potentials, resulting from complex interactions of motor proteins with their molecular tracks (cytoskeleton filaments or nucleic acids), with fuel molecules (ATP or related compounds), with hydrolysis products in different biochemical states, and possibly with other molecules existing in the cellular medium. Because molecular tracks for motor proteins are periodic,

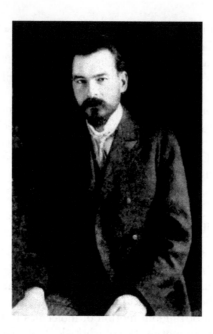

FIGURE 7.1   The famous Polish-Austrian physicist Marian von Smoluchowski (1872–1917) who was one of the pioneers in theoretical studies of Brownian motion, kinetics and stochastic processes in physics, chemistry, and biology. He was a very talented person in many directions. Smoluchowski was not only a great scientist but also an excellent pianist, gifted painter, and advanced mountain climber.

these potentials are also spatially periodic. While moving along each of the potential surfaces, the motor protein merely diffuses in the direction of the local minimum in the free-energy surface; see Fig. 7.3. However, a chemical reaction that involves the molecular motor will typically lead to a stochastic switch to a different biochemical state. This means that the motor hops to another potential surface (Fig. 7.3). It is also important to note that the relative spatial locations of minima in the free-energy potential curves may be shifted. There are, indeed, theoretical arguments suggesting that shifted potentials are more beneficial for the transport of motor proteins (Julicher et al. 1997) [76].

The asymmetry of the potential surfaces is important for deciding in what direction the motor protein prefers to move. It is also the main reason why this approach is called a thermal ratchet. A ratchet (see Fig. 7.4) is widely utilized in various tools and machines: it is a mechanical device that really allows the motion (linear or rotational) in only one direction, while very strongly suppressing the motion in the opposite direction. This analogy is very useful for understanding the dynamics of biological molecular motors. But the asymme-

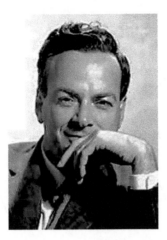

FIGURE 7.2 Richard Feynman (1918–1988) is the famous American physicist and Nobel Prize winner who is also known for his efforts to popularize science and technology. He introduced the idea of "thermal ratchets" that stimulated a development of the continuum potential description for biological molecular motors. What really made Richard Feynman famous were his efforts to popularize science and technology to the general public via lectures, popular books and presentations. The idea of thermal ratchets was presented in popular lectures intended for high school and undergraduate students (Feynman et al. 1966) [52]. Feynman was also one of the first who introduced the concept of nanotechnology.

try in potentials is not enough to support the directed motion of motors. If there is an equilibrium for chemical transitions between different states, the molecular motor will fluctuate around some average position, $\langle x \rangle = const$, where x denotes the position of the particle along its molecular track, with the overall velocity equal to zero,

$$V = \frac{d\langle x \rangle}{dt} = 0. \tag{7.1}$$

It is not possible to have a non-zero velocity for a motor protein at equilibrium since this would imply work done against some external forces (e.g., viscous forces are always present in the cellular environment). It would thus violate the First Law of Thermodynamics since no heat is taken from the outside while the molecular motor could do the work. The important conclusion from this short discussion is that chemical transitions that take the motor from one potential surface to another one must be non-equilibrium, i.e., these transitions must be accompanied by absorbing or releasing chemical energy. The sustained motion of the motor proteins requires a constant flow of energy into the system, which is transformed into the mechanical motion.

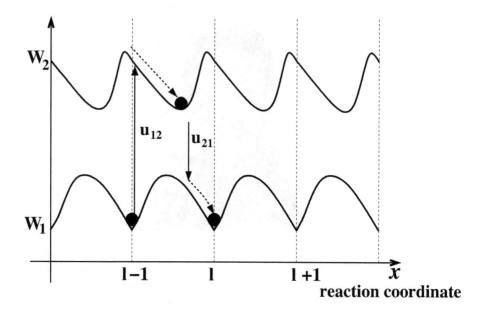

FIGURE 7.3 A schematic view of the transport of motor proteins in continuum thermal ratchet models. Two periodic asymmetric potentials are shown. Solid vertical lines describe stochastic transitions driven by chemical reactions in which molecular motors participate. Dashed lines parallel to potential surfaces correspond to the diffusional motion of molecular motors in the search of the local minima.

Now we can proceed to develop a more explicit analysis of the motor protein's dynamics in thermal ratchet models. One can introduce a function $P_i(x,t)$, which is defined as the probability of finding the molecular motor at the position x at time t while being in the biochemical state i described by the potential surface $W_i(x)$; see Fig. 7.3. This quantity is central for analyzing dynamics of motor proteins using continuum potentials. Its temporal evolution is governed by a set of differential equations which are known as the *Fokker–Planck equations* (Chowdhury 2013, Julicher et al. 1997, Reimann 2002, Xing et al. 2005, Kolomeisky 2013) [30, 76, 131, 183, 82],

$$\frac{\partial P_i(x,t)}{\partial t} + \frac{\partial J_i}{\partial x} = \sum_j u_{ji} P_j(x,t) - \sum_i u_{ij} P_i(x,t). \qquad (7.2)$$

In these expressions, u_{ij} denote the transition rate from the state i to the state j, and J_i is a probability flux along the potential surface W_i. We can easily explain the physical meaning of Fokker-Planck equations using the following arguments. These equations state that the temporal evolution of the probability of finding the motor protein at a specific location is a result of various fluxes in the system. If we forget for a moment about the right side of Eq. (7.2), then it argues the change in the probability is coming from the spatial difference in the fluxes, i.e., from diffusion along the given potential surface. But the molecular motor is also involved in various chemical reactions. So the probability is affected by these processes, and the right side of Eq. (7.2) represents the fluxes from the current biochemical state to other states and from other states to the current state.

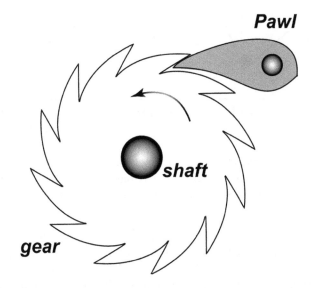

FIGURE 7.4   A schematic picture of the mechanical ratchet device which stimulated the continuum potential description for motor proteins.

The particle current along the reaction coordinate is another important property for analyzing motor proteins dynamics, and it can be found using the following relations (Chowdhury 2013, Julicher et al. 1997, Reimann 2002, Xing et al. 2005, Kolomeisky 2013) [30, 76, 131, 183, 82],

$$J_i(x,t) = \mu_i \left[-k_B T \frac{\partial P_i(x,t)}{\partial x} - P_i(x,t)\frac{\partial W_i(x)}{\partial x} - P_i(x,t)\frac{\partial W_{ext}(x)}{\partial x} \right], \quad (7.3)$$

where a parameter μ_i describes a mobility of the motor protein molecule in the state i. The mobility is directly related with a diffusion constant D_i of the motor protein in the state i,

$$\mu_i = \frac{D_i}{k_B T}. \qquad (7.4)$$

It was also assumed here that some external potential $W_{ext}(x)$ is applied to the system. The Eq. (7.3) states that the particle current consists of three

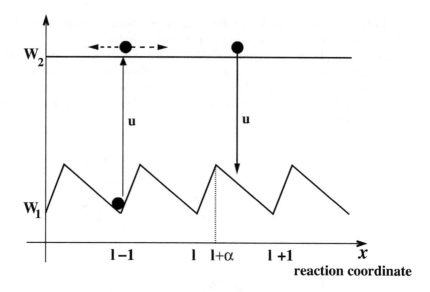

FIGURE 7.5 A simple two-state ratchet potentials model for the motion of motor proteins. The potential $W_1(x)$ is piecewise-linear, while the potential W_2 is flat. The rates of switching between states are the same and equal to u.

terms. The first one is a "concentration gradient" contribution since the flux will appear if the probabilities (concentrations) of motor proteins are not the same at the neighboring spatial positions. While this term is independent of the potential, the second contribution arises due to the action of the potential that obviously changes the probabilities too—the motor particles prefer to be found at the local minima of the potential surface. The last term represents the contribution to the flux created by an external potential.

In order to fully analyze the dynamic behavior of motor proteins using the continuum ratchet potentials approach, one should solve Eqs. (7.2) and (7.3). In some cases it can be done analytically if potential functions are known explicitly. To illustrate the method, let us consider a simple system with two states (two free-energy potential curves) as shown in Fig. 7.5. We assume that the molecular motor can diffuse along the saw-tooth potential $W_1(x)$ or along the flat potential $W_2(x)$. It can switch between the potential surfaces with the same rate u (see Fig. 7.5). The asymmetry of the potential $W_1(x)$ is specified by a parameter $0 \leq \alpha \leq 1$ that shows the relative position of the maximum. The potential is symmetric only for $\alpha = 1/2$. Eqs. (7.2) and (7.3) simplify in the stationary-state limit, and it can be shown that the steady-state flux of molecular motors, $J = J_1 + J_2$, is given by (Ajdari and Prost 1992, Astumian and Bier 1994) [3, 9],

$$J = \frac{u}{4}\left[erf\left(\frac{\alpha\sqrt{u}}{2}\right) - erf\left(\frac{(1-\alpha)\sqrt{u}}{2}\right)\right], \qquad (7.5)$$

where the function $erf(x)$ is known as the *error function*, defined as

$$erf(x) = \frac{2}{\sqrt{\pi}} \int_0^x e^{-y^2} dy. \tag{7.6}$$

One can see from Eq. (7.5) that the particle flux depends on the symmetry of the potential $W_1(x)$. The non-zero current of molecular motors at large times is possible only for asymmetric potential with $\alpha \neq 1/2$.

For more realistic situations with many free-energy surfaces and more complex potential functions analytical solutions of Eqs. (7.2) and (7.3) generally cannot be found, and only numerical calculations can be done. However, some qualitative arguments about motor protein dynamics and their efficiency still can be made (Julicher et al. 1997) [76].

7.3 CRITICAL ANALYSIS

Continuum ratchet potentials have been employed for analyzing motor protein dynamics in several cases (Kolomeisky 2013, Julicher et al. 1997, Xing et al. 2005, Chowdhury 2013) [82, 76, 183, 30]. These chemically driven ratchet models are quite convenient and powerful because they provide a simple and consistent description of dynamic properties of biological molecular motors. The advantages of using Markov–Fokker–Planck models include a physically appealing simple picture of microscopic processes associated with functioning of motor proteins in the cellular environment, and a small number of relevant parameters that describe the system. Continuum potentials methods can be also easily analyzed because they fit well for established mathematical treatments via a variety of analytical and numerical methods. In addition, ratchet models play a very important theoretical role since they serve as a starting point of fundamental studies that probe the nature of non-equilibrium phenomena (Lau et al. 2007, Verley et al. 2011) [91, 176].

At the same time, a critical overview of the main features of continuum ratchet potentials methods suggests that their applications for quantitative modeling of motor proteins and for understanding microscopic mechanisms of their behavior might be problematic (Kolomeisky and Fisher, 2007, Kolomeisky 2013) [84, 82]. As we discussed above, analytical calculations are possible for very few oversimplified and mostly unrealistic situations. The application of ratchet models for real biological systems requires numerical computations that in many cases are quite demanding. The main bottleneck in the successful application of Markov–Fokker–Planck models for biological molecular motors is the exact form of potential functions. This is because explicit estimates of dynamic properties of motor proteins depend on the functional behavior of free-energy potentials. In principle, the potentials can be determined from experimental information such as molecular structures in different conformations, ionic strength of solutions, concentration of relevant molecules, binding/unbinding equilibrium constants, and many other factors. However, in practice, it is almost impossible to derive the potential functions.

As a result, approximations must be used in calculation of dynamic properties of motor proteins, which significantly lowers the usefulness of ratchet models. There is a hope that increasing the amount of the structural information as well as improved computational abilities in full atomic simulations will provide a better estimate for potential functions. But currently the situation is not satisfactory to reliably apply continuum potentials methods for quantitative analysis of mechanisms governing motor proteins. Furthermore, ratchet models are not very flexible in application for systems with complex biochemical networks.

This critical analysis of continuum potential methods implies that ratchet models can be successfully utilized for uncovering qualitative trends in molecular motor dynamics as well as for understanding some general fundamental features of non-equilibrium systems. But the applicability of Markov–Fokker–Planck models for comprehensive quantitative analysis of motor proteins is quite limited, and it is hard to use them for making experimentally testable predictions. So one should be careful in interpretation of results obtained by continuum ratchet potentials for motor protein dynamic properties.

7.4 SUMMARY

In this chapter, we started to discuss theoretical ideas that were proposed for analyzing the mechanisms and functioning of motor proteins. First, we clarified that the role of theoretical models is to provide a fully quantitative connection between dynamic and mechanical properties of biological molecular motors and biochemical processes that control their behavior. In the next step, the fundamental constraints on possible theoretical models for motor proteins were discussed. These limitations are the consequences of the symmetry of the system, and they also result from the requirements that fundamental concepts in physics and chemistry cannot be violated.

We then concentrated on a general description of theoretical methods for understanding biological molecular motors. Two main theoretical ideas currently dominate the field. One of them suggests that the motor protein dynamics can be viewed as a motion in a time-dependent free-energy landscape, while the other approach is based on discrete-state stochastic models. The first approach, which is known as the continuum ratchet potentials method, was fully analyzed in this chapter. The main idea of the method is to consider the motor protein as a particle that travels along these continuum potentials, stochastically transitioning between them. These potentials are the result of complex chemical and physical interactions in the system. To obtain dynamic properties of biological molecular motors, Fokker–Planck equations were presented and explained. It is argued that the particle motion can be observed if transitions between potentials are out of equilibrium. In addition, the role of asymmetry in potential surfaces was discussed. The approach was illustrated by considering a simple two-state ratchet potentials model.

In the end, we presented a critical analysis of thermal ratchet models and their applications to motor proteins. It was suggested that continuum potentials methods can be used for understanding general features of motor protein dynamics, but quantitative description of all features of biological molecular motors cannot be reliably obtained with this approach. The main problem with the method is the determination of potentials, which cannot be done reliably using current theoretical methods and experimental information. But it was argued that this issue might be resolved in the future with improvements in computer simulation techniques and with more detailed experimental observations.

CHAPTER 8

Theory for Motor Proteins: Discrete-State Stochastic Models

CONTENTS

8.1   INTRODUCTION

In the previous chapter we started to analyze theoretical methods proposed for investigating motor proteins functioning in cellular systems. Continuum ratchet potential methods were discussed first. The main idea of this approach is to view dynamics of biological molecular motors as a motion in the effective potentials created by a complex set of chemical and physical interactions in the system. Despite the fact that continuum ratchet models were successful in explaining many features of motor proteins, the application of this approach is rather limited. As we explained, the main reason for this is that it is difficult to properly calculate potentials for ratchet models. In addition, these potentials still cannot be obtained from experiments with a reasonable degree of reliability. But the quantitative power of continuum ratchet models strongly depends on the functional form of the effective free-energy potentials. All these observations stimulated additional efforts in a search for alternative theoretical ideas for studying biological molecular motors.

One of the most important observations about motor proteins is that they are involved in a large number of chemical reactions during their active functioning in cells. First of all, motor proteins are enzymes that accelerate some specific reactions such as the hydrolysis of ATP, polymerization of nucleic acids, and synthesis of proteins. In addition, motor proteins frequently bind/unbind to cytoskeleton filaments or other molecular tracks (nucleic acids, proteins), and they also participate in many other biochemical processes. It is reasonable to suggest that these chemical transformations might be coupled to the dynamics of motor proteins. It was a starting point for developing an alternative theoretical method based on discrete-state stochastic models of traditional chemical kinetics (Qian 2005, Qian and Beard 2008, Kolomeisky and Fisher 2007, Chowdhury 2013, Kolomeisky 2013, Lipowsky and Jaster 2003) [127, 17, 84, 30, 82, 128]. Our aim in this chapter is to fully analyze this theoretical idea.

8.2   DISCRETE-STATE STOCHASTIC APPROACH

8.2.1   *Linear Sequential Models*

The main idea of the discrete-state approach is that the motion of molecular motors can be viewed as a set of chemical transitions between discrete biochemical states that might also have different spatial positions (Fisher and Kolomeisky 1999, Kolomeisky and Fisher 2007, Kolomeisky 2013) [55, 84, 82]. To explain this method we consider first a linear sequential discrete-state stochastic model as presented in Fig. 8.1. The dynamics of a single molecular motor in this system can be explicitly analyzed. Here we assume that all possible biochemical states for the motor protein belong to one path (Fig. 8.1). This also means that the molecular motor bound to the site l along the linear track will go through the whole enzymatic cycle via a sequence of N intermediate states. These states might have different spatial positions (as projected to the linear reaction coordinate; see Fig. 8.1), and it is not necessary for them to be equally separated. The distance between two identical binding sites on the linear track is given by d. It also corresponds to the step size of the molecular motor. For kinesin and dynein motor proteins moving along the microtubules, we have $d = 8.2$ nm, while for myosins V traveling along actin filaments, this distance is larger, $d \simeq 36$ nm. For many nucleic acid motor proteins this length is variable and it can be very short, as small as the distance between the neighboring nucleotides, $d \simeq 0.3$ nm.

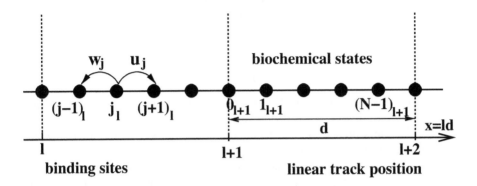

FIGURE 8.1 A schematic view of a linear sequential discrete-state stochastic model for investigating dynamics of single motor proteins. Filled circles in the upper line represent different biochemical states. There are N states per each binding site. Solid horizontal lines between the circles correspond to reversible chemical transitions between states. Vertical dashed lines separate chemical states belonging to different binding positions along the filament. Transition rates u_j and w_j describe forward and backward transitions from the state j. The horizontal line shows the linear track and possible binding sites for the molecular motor. The distance between binding sites is the same and it is equal to d.

Each possible state of the motor protein we label as j_l with $j = 0, 1, \cdots, N-1$, as shown in Fig. 8.1. The label j_l means that the molecular motor is bound to the site l along the linear track, and it is found in the chemical state j. These states describe different stages of the enzymatic process catalyzed by the action of motor proteins. For example, if we consider biological molecular motors that are fueled by the hydrolysis of ATP, then the state 0_l might describe the situation when the motor is bound to the molecular track at the binding site l, awaiting for the arrival of the ATP molecule to be hydrolyzed. The next state 1_l would correspond to the state where ATP together with the motor protein is bound to the linear track at the site l. To be even more specific, let us consider kinesin motor proteins (labeled as K) that translocate along the microtubules (labeled as M) and hydrolyze ATP molecules into ADP and inorganic phosphate that we label as P_i. One could propose the possible simple chemical pathway for the processes associated with kinesins translocating along the microtubules,

$$\text{M} \cdot \text{K} + \text{ATP} \quad \underset{w_1}{\overset{u_0}{\rightleftharpoons}} \quad \text{M} \cdot \text{K} \cdot \text{ATP} \quad \underset{w_1}{\overset{u_1}{\rightleftharpoons}} \quad \text{M} \cdot \text{K} \cdot \text{ADP} \cdot \text{P}_\mathbf{i} \quad \underset{w_3}{\overset{u_2}{\rightleftharpoons}} \quad \text{M} \cdot \text{K} \cdot \text{ADP}$$

$$\underset{w_4}{\overset{u_3}{\rightleftharpoons}} \quad \text{M} \cdot \text{K}. \tag{8.1}$$

This scheme corresponds to the discrete-state sequential stochastic model in Fig. 8.1 with only $N = 4$ intermediate states.

As we mentioned above, each enzymatic cycle has N sequential biochemical states, and the cycle is repeated at every binding site. Then it is clear from this observation that the system is periodic (i.e., all binding sites are identical), reflecting on the important symmetry property of the system. From the state j_l the motor can step forward to the state $(j+1)_l$ with a rate u_j. At the same time, a rate w_j describes the backward transition to the state $(j-1)_l$ (see Fig. 8.1). Because of periodicity, these rates must satisfy the following conditions,

$$u_{j+kN} \equiv u_j, \quad w_{j+kN} \equiv w_j, \tag{8.2}$$

for any integer number k. In addition, it is important to note that in these discrete-state models all chemical transitions between various states are assumed to be reversible. This is consistent with our fundamental arguments on the nature of chemical transformations, and it also agrees with experiments where some of the backward transitions have been directly observed (Kolomeisky and Fisher 2007, Kolomeisky 2013, Carter and Cross 2005, Clancy et al. 2011, Sellers and Veigel 2010) [84, 82, 27, 31, 146]. Furthermore, no assumption about equilibrium in any of the chemical transitions in the system is made.

To fully analyze the linear sequential discrete-state stochastic model from Fig. 8.1 one needs to concentrate on a function $P_j(l, t)$, which is defined as a probability of finding the molecular motor in the state j_l at time t (Kolomeisky and Fisher 2007, Kolomeisky 2013) [84, 82]. This quantity, which is related to a concentration of motor proteins in the given chemical state, is evolving in time according to a differential equation,

$$\frac{dP_j(l, t)}{dt} = u_{j-1} P_{j-1}(l, t) + w_{j+1} P_{j+1}(l, t) - [u_j + w_j] P_j(l, t), \tag{8.3}$$

which is also known as a *master equation*. We already encountered such equations in the Chapter 5 when random walks were introduced. It is relatively easy to understand the physical meaning of the master equation. This is simply a statement of the conservation of the probability. More specifically, the change in the probability of finding the motor protein in the state j_l [the left-hand side of the Eq. (8.3)] has two contributions. One of them is positive, i.e., the probability increases with time, and it comes from two fluxes into the state j_l from the neighboring states $(j-1)_l$ and $(j+1)_l$. It is given by the first two terms on the right-hand side of the Eq. (8.3). The probability decreases with time due to the fluxes out of the state j_l into the forward and backward states; see Fig. 8.1. This negative contribution is represented by the third term on the right-hand side in the Eq. (8.3).

Considering the motion of the single motor protein in the biochemical pathway presented in Fig. 8.1 more closely, we recognize that, strikingly, its dynamics are very similar to a behavior of a random walker that we already discussed in the Chapter 5. Thus the molecular motor can be viewed as the random walker that travels along the periodic one-dimensional infinite lattice of discrete states, which has a period of size N. This is a very important observation since mapping the motion of motor proteins into dynamics of random walkers allows us to use a well-developed mathematical framework [first outlined by B. Derrida in 1983 (Derrida 1983) [40]] that leads to a comprehensive description of all dynamic properties of biological molecular motors (Kolomeisky and Fisher 2007, Kolomeisky 2013) [84, 82]. More specifically, the random-walk approach provides tools to obtain exact and explicit expressions for stationary velocity V and for the mean dispersion (also known as the effective diffusion constant) D (Kolomeisky and Fisher 2007, Kolomeisky 2013) [84, 82]. We can associate $x(t)$ as a position of the molecular motor (monitoring, e.g., the center of mass of the molecule or some other specific position) on the linear track at time t. Then these dynamic properties, V and D, are defined as follows. The steady-state velocity of the motor protein is given by

$$V = V(\{u_j, w_j\}) = \lim_{t \to \infty} \frac{d\langle x(t) \rangle}{dt}. \tag{8.4}$$

In other words, the velocity is equal to the average slope of many motor protein trajectories at large times. This is the way to determine it in experiments. Similarly, the effective diffusion constant is written as

$$D = D(\{u_j, w_j\}) = \frac{1}{2} \lim_{t \to \infty} \frac{d}{dt} \left[\langle x^2(t) \rangle - \langle x(t) \rangle^2 \right]. \tag{8.5}$$

The mean dispersion can be obtained in experiments as the average slope obtained at large t by looking into the mean-square displacements as a function of time for the molecular motor's motion.

To illustrate how we explicitly calculate these dynamic properties, let us start with the simplest sequential discrete-state model that has $N = 1$. This is the case when the enzymatic cycle has only one chemical state, and the binding sites coincide with these states. Clearly, this is an oversimplified and probably unrealistic situation with regard to the motor proteins. It can be shown (see derivations in the Mathematical Appendix) that

$$V = d(u_0 - w_0), \quad D = \frac{d^2}{2}(u_0 + w_0), \tag{8.6}$$

for the average velocity and dispersion, respectively. Recall that d is the motor protein step-size that corresponds to the distance between neighboring binding sites. These results are exactly the same as were found for the continuous-time random walker and given in Eq. (5.64). More complex and more realistic is the situation with two chemical states per each cycle, i.e., for $N = 2$. In this case the expression for the mean velocity is given by (see the Mathematical Appendix),

$$V = d\frac{u_0 u_1 - w_0 w_1}{u_0 + w_0 + u_1 + w_1},\tag{8.7}$$

while for the effective diffusion constant

$$D = \frac{d^2}{2}\frac{(u_0 u_1 + w_0 w_1) - 2(V/d)^2}{u_0 + w_0 + u_1 + w_1}.\tag{8.8}$$

Generally, as shown in the Mathematical Appendix, one can compute velocities and dispersions for the periodic linear sequential discrete-state model with *any* N and for an *arbitrary* set of chemical transition rates u_j and w_j. This is the important observation since it provides a direct coupling between dynamic properties of motor proteins, which are measured in single-molecule experiments, with chemical rates that can be obtained *independently* from bulk chemical kinetic experiments. From this point of view, the discrete stochastic method is much more convenient than the continuum ratchets approach since the input parameters here are derived from other experiments, in contrast to potentials that must be computed.

Another significant advantage of the discrete-state stochastic models is the ability to explicitly calculate *all* dynamic properties of biological molecular motors. This leads to a better understanding of mechanisms that govern their activities. For example, one can introduce a function called *randomness*, which is defined as

$$r = \frac{2D}{dV}.\tag{8.9}$$

It is a quantity that can be evaluated from experimental measurements with a reasonable degree of precision (Kolomeisky and Fisher 2007, Svoboda and Block 1994, Schnitzer et al. 2000) [84, 159, 142]. It was argued, using the discrete-state stochastic picture, that it measures the degree of dynamic fluctuations in the moving motor proteins. In addition, it was proved mathematically that for the linear sequential discrete models it obeys the inequality, $r \geq 1/N$ (Koza 2002) [87]. This can be seen if we take all forward rates to be the same, $u_j = u$ and all backward rates to disappear, $w_j = 0$. Then one can show that $r = 1/N$, because this corresponds to the case of $N = 1$ but with the step size equal to d/N. Obviously, taking into account the backward rates should only increase the fluctuations for single molecular motors, i.e., the randomness must be higher than the limiting value. For example, experiments on kinesin motor proteins at large concentrations of ATP suggest that $r \simeq 0.39$ (Visscher et al. 1999) [177]. This means that there are, at least, three ATP-independent intermediate chemical transitions ($r > 1/3$), in which the kinesin actively participate. This agrees with the simple chemical kinetic scheme presented in Eq. (8.1). Now, if we have experimentally measured randomness parameters and explicit formulas for V and D, then this significantly narrows the range of possible models that could describe the system. This is a good illustration of how discrete-state stochastic models might be useful for obtaining the valuable information on mechanisms of motor proteins.

8.2.2 *Forces in Motor Proteins*

The discrete-state stochastic approach is very powerful in explaining various microscopic properties of biological molecular motors. For example, the motor proteins catalyze some specific biochemical processes (hydrolysis of ATP or related compounds, polymerization of nucleic acids, and synthesis of proteins), and the fraction of the energy released during these processes is utilized by the motor to develop forces (for linear motors) or torques (for rotary motors). In the discrete-state stochastic method these driving forces can be explicitly estimated, providing another way of clarifying mechanisms of motor proteins (Fisher and Kolomeisky 1999) [55].

The following arguments can be presented to explain the forces exerted by motor proteins. It can be shown for the linear sequential model in Fig. 8.1 that the force developed by the molecular motor is equal to

$$F_S = \frac{k_B T}{d} \ln \prod_{j=0}^{N-1} \left(\frac{u_j}{w_j} \right). \tag{8.10}$$

This force can be viewed as a chemical driving force since it is a result of difference in the chemical potentials for products (after completing one enzymatic cycle) and reactants (before the enzymatic cycle). We can understand this simple result if we recall the connection between thermodynamics and chemical kinetics. Let us consider a process that consists of the motor protein moving from one binding site to the next one. In terms of the linear sequential model in Fig. 8.1, it corresponds to the set of transitions that starts at the state 0_l and finishes at the state 0_{l+1}. There are N sequential chemical transitions in this process. One could estimate the equilibrium constant K_{eq} for the motor protein stepping between neighboring binding sites. If we have only one transition, $N = 1$, then the equilibrium constant can be easily written as $K_{eq} = \frac{u_0}{w_0}$. For the sequential process with $N > 1$ intermediate states this result can be easily generalized, producing

$$K_{eq} = \prod_{j=0}^{N-1} \left(\frac{u_j}{w_j} \right). \tag{8.11}$$

But the equilibrium constant is directly related to the free-energy change occurring in the process. Thus, the expression

$$\Delta G_0 = -k_B T \ln K_{eq} \tag{8.12}$$

gives the amount of the free energy that is released when the motor protein completes one enzymatic cycle and moves one step forward a distance d along the linear track (Fig. 8.1). This free-energy difference is due to the enzymatic process, and, in principle, all of this energy can be converted into mechanical motion. If one applies the external force F_{ext} that opposes the motion of the motor protein, then the work done by the motor can be written as $W = F_{ext}d$. This suggests that the maximal external force $F_{ext,max}$ can be easily evaluated as

$$F_{ext,max} = F_S = -\frac{\Delta G_0}{d}. \tag{8.13}$$

This force is known as a *stall force*. It is equal to the external force that must be applied to stop the motor from moving forward. In the linear sequential model from the Fig. 8.1, this situation corresponds exactly to a chemical equilibrium. The motor protein sits, on average, at one specific binding site, and its mean drift velocity is zero. However, it might not be the case in other more general discrete-state stochastic models with complex biochemical pathways (Kolomeisky 2013) [82].

From these explanations about the forces exerted by the motor proteins we can make one important conclusion. It is not possible to neglect *any* of the backward transitions in the system. To see this, let us assume that, at least, one of these transition rates is assumed to be equal zero, $w_j = 0$. Then from Eqs. (8.10) and (8.13) one would predict that the exerted force or the free-energy difference is infinite, which is clearly unphysical since it violates the First and Second Laws of Thermodynamics. There will be no force in the universe that can stop such a motor. This motor would be able to do an infinite amount of work without consuming much heat. This discussion again supports our arguments that all chemical processes associated with motor proteins must be considered as reversible, even if experimentally some of them are not yet observed. Clearly, violating this condition does not allow us to understand properly the microscopic mechanisms in biological molecular motors.

During their functioning in cells, motor proteins are affected by various external forces and fields. Discrete-state stochastic models provide a convenient method of accounting for the effect of external loads and fields in biological molecular motors. We already discussed in Chapter 4 how the external force modifies the equilibrium constant for any chemical process. For the motor protein stepping along its linear track against the force F it leads to

$$K_{eq}(F) = K_{eq}(F = 0) \exp\left(-\frac{Fd}{k_B T}\right). \tag{8.14}$$

Then Eq. (8.11) suggests that every transition rate might be affected by the external force. The possible behavior of chemical rates can be described by introducing new parameters $\theta_j^{\pm}$ known as *load-distribution factors* (Fisher and Kolomeisky 1999, Kolomeisky and Fisher 2007, Kolomeisky 2013) [55, 84, 82],

$$u_j(F) = u_j(0) \exp(-\theta_j^+ Fd/k_B T), \quad w_j(F) = w_j(0) \exp(\theta_j^- Fd/k_B T), \tag{8.15}$$

with the additional requirement that

$$\sum_{j=0}^{N-1} (\theta_j^+ + \theta_j^-) = 1. \tag{8.16}$$

To understand the physical meaning of these parameters, let us consider a simple model with $N = 1$. Then the potential energy surfaces for the process affected by the external force and for the scenario without force are presented in Fig. 8.2. When the external load is activated, the work $W = Fd$ is done by the motor and the free-energy energy at the end of the reaction must be modified by this amount. This change obviously should affect both the forward and the backward reactions; see Fig. 8.2. However, we do not know how, so we introduce parameters θ^+ and θ^- to phenomenologically quantify this effect. This means that the relative energy of the state 0 is lower by $\theta^+ Fd$, while the energy for the state 1 increases by $\theta^- Fd$ when the external load is switched on. The conservation of energy requires that $(\theta^+ + \theta^-)Fd = Fd$. Now, recalling that the rate of the chemical reaction is proportional to the exponent of the energy barrier, we conclude that the forward reaction is modified under the effect of external force,

$$u(F) = u(F = 0) \exp(-\theta^+ Fd/k_B T). \tag{8.17}$$

Similarly, we can show for the backward rate,

$$w(F) = w(F = 0) \exp(\theta^- Fd/k_B T). \tag{8.18}$$

These arguments can be easily extended to general linear sequential stochastic models from Fig. 8.1, justifying the use of Eqs. (8.15) and (8.16).

The load-distribution factors $\theta_j^{\pm}$ also provide important mechanistic information about the motor protein activities. The maxima and minima in the free-energy landscape for dynamics of molecular motors correspond to the products $\theta_j^{\pm} d$. For example, $\theta_j^+ d$ gives the distance (along the reaction coordinate) between the state j and the transition activated complex (the top of the barrier) for the chemical process to go to the state $j + 1$. Correspondingly, $(\theta_j^+ + \theta_{j+1}^-)d$ is the distance between the states j and $j + 1$. This analysis also defines the concept of substeps. Then one might conclude that the spatial position of intermediate states might differ significantly, so they might be seen directly in experiments. This is a very important theoretical prediction of the discrete-state stochastic models since the substeps have been observed in single-molecule studies of several motor protein systems (Kolomeisky and Fisher 2007) [84].

The application of the load-distribution factors is a powerful tool for studying mechanisms of motor proteins, but one should remember that this is not exact (Kolomeisky 2013) [82]. Our explanations of the microscopic origin of $\theta_j^{\pm}$ using the Fig. 8.2 implicitly assumed that the position and the energy of the transition-state complex (the top of the free-energy curve) are not affected by the external forces. As a result, the load-distribution parameters

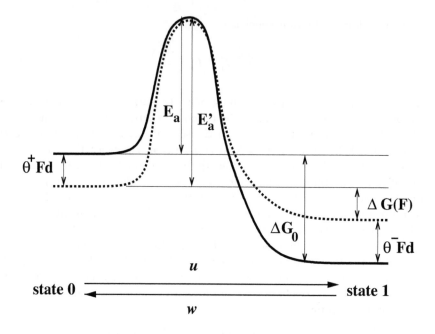

FIGURE 8.2   A schematic view of the free-energy profile for a simple linear sequential model for $N = 1$ with the forward rate u and the backward rate w. The solid curve describes the reaction in the absence of the external force. The dotted curve is the free-energy profile under the effect of the external force F. ΔG_0 and $\Delta G(F)$ are the free-energy differences for the process without the force and with the force, respectively. E_a and E'_a are energy barriers for the forward reaction without and with the external force, respectively.

are taken to be force-independent. This might be a reasonable picture if the absolute values of energy barriers are much larger than the changes to the free energy due to the work against the external force F, i.e., for $E_a \gg Fd$. In other words, for slow chemical transitions (large barriers) the use of force-independent load-distribution factors is acceptable, while for fast chemical reactions (small barriers) it might not provide a correct description of the dynamics. It seems that for many protein systems that are currently investigated this approximation works quite well. However, there are indications that for some chemical processes in biopolymers, such simplified theoretical models might lead to fundamentally wrong results (Walcott 2008, Makarov 2013) [178, 104]. Thus we should be careful in the interpretation of the mechanisms of motor proteins using the concept of load-distribution factors. It is a very powerful tool, but one should always remember these fundamental limitations.

8.2.3 Dwell Times and First-Passage Analysis

In many single-molecule experiments the residence times of biological molecular motors in different spatial positions, corresponding to specific biochemical states of motor proteins, are measured with a high temporal resolution (Mehta et al. 1999, Nishiyama et al. 2002, Carter and Cross 2005) [110, 99, 27]. These parameters are called *dwell times*, and they are frequently utilized for understanding dynamics of motor proteins (Kolomeisky and Fisher 2007, Kolomeisky 2013) [84, 82]. The discrete-state stochastic model is a powerful method that can help us to analyze dwell times and couple them with microscopic properties of molecular motors. Because the single motors in this theoretical approach can be viewed as random walkers, we immediately associate the observed transitions and dwell times with the concept of first-passage processes which was discussed in detail in the Chapter 5. It is clear that the full distribution of dwell times (or first-passage times) contains full information on mechanisms of motor proteins. The method of first-passage events allows us to apply a well-developed mathematical analysis to explicitly evaluate dynamic properties of biological molecular motors (Kolomeisky and Fisher 2007, Kolomeisky 2013, Kolomeisky and Fisher 2003, Kolomeisky et al. 2005) [84, 82, 83, 85].

To illustrate the application of the first-passage techniques for motor proteins in the discrete-state stochastic approach, let us consider again the linear sequential model in Fig. 8.1. We are interested in understanding the distribution of transition events that start at some state j and finish in the state N, and how it can be coupled to microscopic chemical rates for molecular motors. One can introduce a function $F_{j,N}(t)$ defined as a probability of reaching the state N for the first time at time t if the molecular motor started at $t = 0$ at the state j. These distribution functions change with time, and their temporal evolution can be described by *backward master equations* (Kolomeisky 2013) [82],

$$\frac{dF_{j,N}(t)}{dt} = u_j F_{j+1,N}(t) + w_j F_{j-1,N}(t) - [u_j + w_j]F_{j,N}(t). \qquad (8.19)$$

As we already discussed in the Chapter 5, these equations, although similar to ordinary master equations, differ from them in many aspects. The main reason for this is that different quantities are analyzed. The ordinary master equations describe changes in the probability of finding the particle at the specific state, while the backward master equation controls the probability of reaching the specific state from the known starting position. In many cases, Eq. (8.19) can be solved exactly and it provides a comprehensive description of the motor protein dynamics (Kolomeisky 2013, Chowdhury 2013, Kolomeisky and Fisher 2003, Kolomeisky et al. 2005, Tsygankov et al. 2007) [82, 30, 83, 167]. The solutions for the linear sequential model with $N = 2$ are given in the Mathematical Appendix.

Suppose we want to understand the stepping dynamics in the motor protein system that can be described by the linear sequential discrete-state model with N intermediate states. We can then associate the forward steps with transitions from the state 0_l to the state $N_l \equiv 0_{l+1}$, while the backward steps correspond to the transition from 0_l to $(-N)_l \equiv 0_{l-1}$; see Fig. 8.1. To describe the forward steps in this system we employ the first-passage probability function $F_{0,N}(t)$ to reach the state N for the first time at time t *before* reaching the state $(-N)$. This is the probability of making the forward step before the motor can jump backward, and it correctly describes typical measurements in single-molecule experiments. Similarly, for the backward step we use the function $F_{0,-N}(t)$, the probability of reaching for the first time the state $(-N)$ starting from the state 0, but before reaching the state N. One can introduce parameters Π_+ and Π_- defined as probabilities to make the forward or the backward step, respectively,

$$\Pi_+ = \int_0^\infty F_{0,N}(t)dt, \quad \Pi_- = \int_0^\infty F_{0,-N}(t)dt. \tag{8.20}$$

They are also known as *splitting probabilities*. Similarly, τ_+ and τ_- are mean dwell times before the forward and backward steps, respectively. These quantities are defined as

$$\tau_+ = \frac{\int_0^\infty tF_{0,N}(t)dt}{\Pi_+}, \quad \tau_- = \frac{\int_0^\infty tF_{0,-N}(t)dt}{\Pi_-}. \tag{8.21}$$

It is also important to note that the first-passage properties of motor proteins are directly connected to their dynamic properties. For example, for the mean stepping velocity it can be shown that (Kolomeisky et al. 2005) [85]

$$V = d\frac{(\Pi_+ - \Pi_-)}{\tau_+}. \tag{8.22}$$

Exact calculations of the dwell times for the linear sequential discrete model lead to a very surprising result (Kolomeisky et al. 2005) [85]: the dwell times before the forward and backward steps, τ_+ and τ_- correspondingly, are the same for the motor proteins in the linear sequential model from Fig. 8.1. For the simplest case with $N = 1$ one can see that the splitting probabilities are just the probabilities to go in the forward or in the backward direction,

$$\Pi_+ = \frac{\frac{u_0}{w_0}}{1 + \frac{u_0}{w_0}} = \frac{u_0}{u_0 + w_0}, \quad \Pi_- = \frac{1}{1 + \frac{u_0}{w_0}} = \frac{w_0}{u_0 + w_0}. \tag{8.23}$$

The dwell times in this case are also quite simple to understand,

$$\tau_+ = \tau_- = \frac{1}{u_0 + w_0}. \tag{8.24}$$

They are equal to the total residence time in the state 0. For $N = 2$ the calculations can be done (see the Mathematical Appendix) to show that the splitting probabilities are equal to

$$\Pi_+ = \frac{\frac{u_0 u_1}{w_0 w_1}}{1 + \frac{u_0 u_1}{w_0 w_1}} = \frac{u_0 u_1}{u_0 u_1 + w_0 w_1}, \quad \Pi_- = \frac{1}{1 + \frac{u_0 u_1}{w_0 w_1}} = \frac{w_0 w_1}{u_0 u_1 + w_0 w_1}, \tag{8.25}$$

while for the dwell times the results are

$$\tau_+ = \tau_- = \frac{u_0 + u_1 + w_0 + w_1}{u_0 u_1 + w_0 w_1}. \qquad (8.26)$$

One would naively expect that the times before the forward steps and before the backward steps to be different because under normal conditions in cells the motor protein mostly moves in one direction. How can we understand this unexpected result? Let us look again at the $N = 1$ model. In this case, the dwell times are equal to the residence time of the motor protein at the site 0. But the residence time does not depend on the direction in which the particle will go. The mean lifetime is equal to the inverse of the total rate out of the site, $\tau = 1/(u_0 + w_0)$. Effectively, the dwell times measure the times between *any* stepping events, independently of the direction. Then the average forward and backward stepping times must be the same. At the same time, the probabilities of the forward and backward motions are different. For this reason, the motor protein preferentially moves in one direction. These arguments can be extended to linear sequential models of any size N.

It is also interesting to analyze the splitting probabilities that determine in which direction the motor protein proceeds. It can be shown generally for the linear sequential model with N intermediate states that (Kolomeisky et al. 2005) [85]

$$\Pi_+ = \frac{\prod_{j=0}^{N-1}\left(\frac{u_j}{w_j}\right)}{1 + \prod_{j=0}^{N-1}\left(\frac{u_j}{w_j}\right)}, \quad \Pi_- = \frac{1}{1 + \prod_{j=0}^{N-1}\left(\frac{u_j}{w_j}\right)}. \qquad (8.27)$$

Now we can recall Eqs. (8.11) and (8.12), and these probabilities can be rewritten as

$$\Pi_+ = \frac{\exp\left[-\frac{\Delta G_0}{k_B T}\right]}{1 + \exp\left[-\frac{\Delta G_0}{k_B T}\right]}, \quad \Pi_- = \frac{1}{1 + \exp\left[-\frac{\Delta G_0}{k_B T}\right]}, \qquad (8.28)$$

where ΔG_0 is the free-energy difference for making one step forward. This suggests that splitting probabilities can be explained using thermodynamic arguments. All binding sites 0_l can be divided in two groups: the sites to which the motor came after the forward motion—let us label them as A states; and the sites where the motor came after the backward step - we call them B states. Thus, our system can be viewed as an effective two-state model. All forward steps correspond to a transition from B to A, while the reversed transition describes all backward steps. From this point of view, Π_+ is the probability of finding the system in the state A, while Π_- gives the probability of being in the B state. Obviously, at large times the equilibrium is reached in this effective two-state system. The probabilities of finding the system in the state A or in the state B must be described by a Boltzmann distribution, as we discussed in the Chapter 4. Eq. (8.28) is exactly the Boltzmann distribution for this two-state model.

The application of the method of first-passage events turned out to be very effective for understanding microscopic properties of biological molecular motors. In Fig. 8.3 the results of using the method for myosin-V motor proteins are presented. These proteins move along actin filaments making steps of $d \simeq 36$ nm. The theoretical analysis provided a comprehensive description of the dynamics for myosin-V molecules at all external forces and for different ATP concentrations.

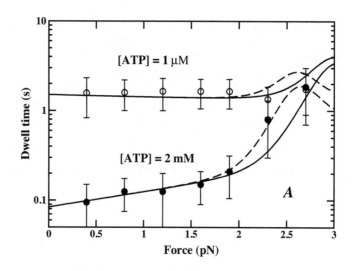

FIGURE 8.3 Mean dwell times of myosin-V motor proteins as a function of external forces at different ATP concentrations. Symbols are experimental measurements from Mehta et al. 1999 [110]. Solid curves are theoretical fits obtained via the first-passage analysis. Dashed curves are theoretical predictions obtained via the first-passage analysis along with assuming step-size fluctuations. The figure is adopted with permission from Kolomeisky and Fisher 2003 [83].

8.2.4 Efficiency of Motor Proteins

As we discussed at the beginning of the book, motor proteins can be viewed as nanoscale engines that transport different molecular species inside of the biological cells. Their behavior is similar to cars and engines that we use in our everyday life. The fuel for molecular motors comes from the chemical reactions that they catalyze. One of the most important characteristics of macroscopic machines is their efficiency, which is defined as (Atkins and de Paula 2009)

[10],

$$\eta = \frac{(-W)}{Q}, \qquad (8.29)$$

where $(-W)$ corresponds to the work done by the system, and Q is the heat provided into the system. Classical thermodynamics gives us an upper bound for the conversion of heat into the work for macroscopic machines. For heat engines that take energy at the temperature T_2 and deliver the work at the lower temperature T_1 it was shown that the maximal efficiency is (Atkins and de Paula 2009) [10]

$$\eta_{max} = \frac{T_2 - T_1}{T_2}. \qquad (8.30)$$

This is known as a *Carnot cycle analysis*. The important conclusion here is that no engine working in equilibrium ever reaches 100% efficiency. For example, if $T_2 = 400$ K and $T_1 = 300$ K, the maximum efficiency is only 25%. In reality it will be even less because of possible losses of energy due to friction and other dissipation. Another more practical quantity to characterize the engines is power, P, which is defined as a work or heat produced per unit of time (Atkins and de Paula 2009) [10].

As an example, let us estimate the efficiency of some motor proteins that experimentally are well investigated: a kinesin hydrolyze 1 ATP molecule when it makes an 8-nm step forward. The input heat is equal to the energy of the chemical reaction of ATP hydrolysis. Schematically, this reaction be written in the simplified way as

$$ATP \rightleftharpoons ADP + P_i. \qquad (8.31)$$

The free energy of this process is given by

$$\Delta G = \Delta G_0 + k_B T \ln \frac{[ADP][P_i]}{[ATP]}, \qquad (8.32)$$

where ΔG_0 is a standard free energy for the process, i.e., when all concentrations are the same and equal to 1 M. The standard free energy has been measured in experiments, and it is estimated as $\Delta G_0 \sim 30 - 35$ kJ/mole or $12 - 14 \, k_B T$ of energy is released after hydrolyzing 1 ATP molecule (Howard 2001) [68]. But we need the total free energy because at typical cellular conditions the second term in Eq. (8.32) is not zero. It is known that in cells $[ATP] \approx [P_i] = 1$ mM and $[ADP] \simeq 10 \, \mu$M (Howard 2001) [68]. Substituting these data into Eq. (8.32) leads us to the estimate that approximately 25 $k_B T$ of energy is available from the ATP hydrolysis. The maximal force (stall force) for kinesin is $\simeq 7$ pN (Visscher et al. 1999, Schnitzer et al. 1999) [177, 142]. The work that kinesin can produce against this stall force is $W = 56$ pN×nm (these strange units are sometimes used because in single-molecule experiments forces are measured in pN and distances are measured in nm), which is equal to $\simeq 14 \, k_B T$. Thus the efficiency of kinesins is close to 56%. Even more efficient are myosin-V motor proteins which also hydrolyze 1 ATP per forward step. They make long steps, $d = 36$ nm, and their stall force is close to 2.5

pN (Mehta et al. 1999) [110]. So the maximal work produced by myosins-V is $W = 22.5\ k_BT$, which gives an efficiency close to 90%! This is a very impressive result since for typical car engines that we use in our machines the efficiency is never above 10%.

Thermodynamic arguments using the Carnot cycle cannot be directly applied to motor proteins that function under non-equilibrium isothermal conditions. Although the efficiency of the molecular motor is maximal at the stalling conditions, the motor protein does not move so it is not a convenient measure of the efficiency. A different theoretical approach to analyze the efficiency of biological molecular motors is needed (Seifert 2001, Golubeva et al. 2012) [145, 117]. To illustrate these arguments, let us consider a motor protein system that can be described by the linear sequential discrete model from Fig. 8.1. It is assumed that the motor operates against the external force $F > 0$. During one cycle the molecular motor makes a step d forward to the next binding site. Then the motor protein obtains the heat from the chemical processes given by

$$Q = F_S d, \tag{8.33}$$

where F_S is the chemical force exerted by the motor [see Eq. (8.10)]. At the same time, the motor produces the work against the external force, $W = -Fd$. The free energy change in the system after one cycle is equal then

$$-\Delta G = Q + W. \tag{8.34}$$

The input power can be estimated then as

$$P_{in} = F_S V = F_S d\, \frac{(\Pi_+ - \Pi_-)}{\tau}, \tag{8.35}$$

where Eq. (8.22) was used to describe the stationary-state velocity V of the motor protein via the splitting probabilities $\Pi_{\pm}$ and the average dwell time τ. Employing the relations between $\Pi_{\pm}$ and the free-energy change after one cycle, we can obtain

$$P_{in} = \frac{F_S d}{\tau} \frac{\left(\exp\left[-\frac{\Delta G_0}{k_B T}\right] - 1\right)}{\left(\exp\left[-\frac{\Delta G_0}{k_B T}\right] + 1\right)}. \tag{8.36}$$

The power that the motor protein delivered can be estimated in the same way,

$$P_{out} = FV = Fd\, \frac{(\Pi_+ - \Pi_-)}{\tau} = \frac{Fd}{\tau} \frac{\left(\exp\left[-\frac{\Delta G_0}{k_B T}\right] - 1\right)}{\left(\exp\left[-\frac{\Delta G_0}{k_B T}\right] + 1\right)}. \tag{8.37}$$

The efficiency is defined then as

$$\eta \equiv \frac{P_{out}}{P_{in}} = \frac{F}{F_S}. \tag{8.38}$$

One can see that the efficiency of the motor protein, in contrast to macroscopic machines, is not bounded and it can reach a unity, i.e., all heat from the catalyzed chemical reaction can be transformed into the work. But the efficiency $\eta = 1$ is reached only at stall conditions ($F = F_S$) where the molecular motor does not move ($V = 0$) and the power output is zero. When we buy a new car we are interested in its performance when it drives, not when it sits in the garage! For this reason, it is more interesting to analyze the non-zero output power for the motor proteins. It varies with changing external forces. The results are presented in Fig. 8.4 for the simple linear sequential discrete model with $N = 1$. The power delivered by the motor protein shows a non-monotonic behavior. It is very small for a weak external force ($F \ll 1$), it starts to grow for intermediate forces reaching the maximal value, and then it decreases to zero at the stalling force; see Fig. 8.4. The power produced by the motor also strongly depends on the load-distribution factors. The strongest power output is observed for small $\theta \approx 0$ (where $\theta_0^+ \equiv \theta$), while for large values ($\theta \approx 1$) the produced power quickly diminishes. These results indicate that molecular motors are much more efficient machines when the transition states for associated chemical processes are closer to the reactants. It is interesting that the analysis of experimental data suggests that for some proteins, such as kinesins and myosins, the load distribution factors are indeed small, indicating that these motors probably operate near the maximum power. However, this conclusion depends on the assumption that motor proteins can be described by the linear sequential discrete-state models as in Fig. 8.1, while experiments show that for many molecular motors more complex biochemical networks are needed (Baker et al. 2004, Clancy et al. 2011) [14, 31].

8.2.5 Discrete-State Stochastic Models for Systems with Complex Biochemical Pathways

A major advantage of the discrete-state stochastic approach is its versatility and flexibility in handling motor protein systems with more complex biochemical pathways. In many instances, experiments indicate that the underlying network of chemical states that support the activities of molecular motors strongly deviate from the simple linear chains discussed so far (Baker et al. 2004, Clancy et al. 2011) [14, 31]. The more realistic picture of the topology of biochemical networks for motor proteins includes multiple parallel pathways, loops, branches, and effectively irreversible detachments. Several examples of discrete-state stochastic models with complex biochemical networks are shown in Fig. 8.5. However, despite the increased complexity, the original Derrida method can still be extended for calculating exactly all dynamic properties of molecular motors in these systems (Kolomeisky 2001, Stukalin and Kolomeisky 2006, Das and Kolomeisky 2008, Kolomeisky 2011, Kolomeisky and Fisher 2007, Kolomeisky 2013) [80, 157, 37, 81, 84, 82]. This allows us to investigate and to understand many important features of mo-

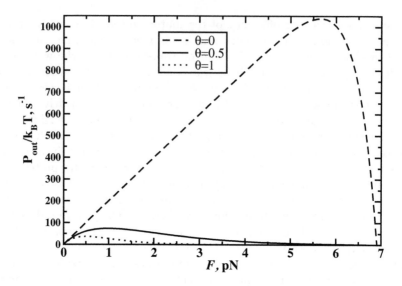

FIGURE 8.4 Output power produced by a single motor protein in the linear sequential discrete-state stochastic model as a function of the external force for different load-distribution factors. Parameters are: $N = 1$, $u = 100$ s^{-1}, $w = 10^4$ s^{-1}, and $d = 8$ nm. The output power is in units of $k_B T$. The dashed curve corresponds to $\theta = 0$, the solid curve is for $\theta = 0.5$ and the dotted curve is for $\theta = 1$.

tor proteins, including the role of spatial fluctuations in myosins-V (Das and Kolomeisky 2008) [37] and the mechanisms of enzymatic action in motor proteins (Kolomeisky 2011) [81].

8.3 CRITICAL ANALYSIS

The main success of the discrete-state stochastic method is a development of the comprehensive and explicit theoretical framework for quantifying all features of motor proteins and their activities. It provides exact analytical expressions for all dynamic properties of biological molecular motors. In addition, discrete-state stochastic models directly couple chemical processes in motor proteins with their dynamic properties, providing a microscopic view of molecular motors functioning. They are also convenient for explaining the effect of external fields. Furthermore, the discrete-state models are powerful tools for understanding the details of how the heat of enzymatically catalyzed chemical reactions is transformed into the mechanical work. It seems that this theoretical approach can account for all available experimental observations ranging from bulk chemical kinetics to single-molecule microscopy.

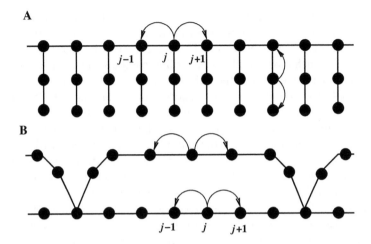

FIGURE 8.5 A schematic view of discrete-state stochastic models for systems with complex biochemical pathways. Solid circles correspond to biochemical states, while solid lines describe possible chemical transitions. (A) The model with branched states. (B) The model with two parallel pathways.

The discrete-state stochastic models have already been successfully applied to analyze several motor proteins including kinesins, myosins, dyneins, RNA and DNA polymerases, ribosomes, and many other systems (Kolomeisky and Fisher 2007, Kolomeisky 2013, Chowdhury 2013) [84, 82, 30].

Although the discrete-state approach seems to describe the motor protein dynamics reasonably well, giving us many clues on underlying molecular mechanisms, there are several limitations of this method that should be discussed. First of all, this method is a phenomenological approach that is not derived from any fundamental theory. It means that if we know the free-energy landscape for the system and all kinetic rates, the dynamic properties of molecular motor can be well predicted. But the microscopic origin of this landscape and why these kinetic rates have specific values is beyond the reach of this approach. We understand that the free-energy profiles and chemical rates are the result of complex interactions in the system. However, the discrete-state models do not provide us with any way to directly estimate these quantities. In addition, the method does not accurately connect dynamic properties of motor proteins with their molecular structures. This significantly limits our abilities to uncover mechanisms of biological molecular motors. Another weak point of discrete models is that a large number of parameters are needed to fully describe dynamic behavior of motor proteins. This complicates the reliable fittings of the experimental observations, which does not help in identifying the correct picture of how motor proteins function. Frequently, several very different models can reproduce the same experimental observations.

Despite these limitations, the discrete-state stochastic models are still much superior to continuum potential methods (see the Chapter 7) in analyzing motor proteins behavior. The main reason is that the discrete-state approach is much more flexible in handling complex biochemical systems, and it is also much better connected with experiments. However, one should notice here that both theoretical ideas proposed for explaining activities of biological molecular motors (the continuum ratchet approach and the discrete-state stochastic method) are related to each other. One can easily see this if we associate the minima in the continuum potential surface with the discrete chemical states. This suggests that at the mathematical level both methods are comparable. However, it seems that the discrete-state models are more convenient in their applications because of closer connections to experiments. It is important to continue to use both theoretical concepts for analyzing general features of motor proteins since they provide a complementary picture for these complex biological systems. At the same, a quantitative description of single-molecule experiments on molecular motors requires the application of the discrete-state stochastic approach.

8.4 SUMMARY

In this chapter we discussed another important theoretical concept for understanding the mechanisms of motor proteins. It is based on the discrete-state stochastic analysis of chemical and mechanical processes associated with molecular motors. In this theoretical method, the motion of motor proteins is described as a set of transitions between discrete biochemical states that can also have different spatial locations.

The main features of the discrete-state stochastic approach were presented using linear sequential models. It was shown how to compute explicitly all dynamic properties of the system by solving master equations. The method was illustrated by calculating velocities and diffusion constants for several simple stochastic models. We then analyzed the forces developed by the active motor proteins as well as their responses to external loads and fields. In order to better understand single-molecule experiments, dwell times of molecular motors in various biochemical states were discussed. The connection between first-passage features and dynamic properties of biological molecular were quantitatively explained. In addition, we evaluated the efficiency of motor proteins as nanoscale engines, and concluded that at typical cellular conditions, molecular motors can be more efficient than the macroscopic equilibrium machines. Furthermore, the flexibility of the discrete-state approach in analyzing motor protein systems with complex biochemical networks of states was discussed.

Finally, we presented a critical evaluation of discrete-state stochastic models. Although these ideas are successfully employed in explaining dynamic properties of various motor protein systems, there are limitations due to weak coupling with molecular structures and with more fundamental concepts. The application of both theoretical methods, continuum ratchets and discrete-state, for motor proteins was compared and analyzed. It was argued that both methods are intrinsically related. We also suggest that the discrete-state methods are much more powerful and convenient in deciphering mechanisms of biological molecular motors because of their close connections to experiments. However, both methods are encouraged to be utilized because they lead to a more comprehensive description of complex mechanochemical processes in motor proteins. But the quantitative nature of single-molecule measurements requires discrete-state stochastic analysis.

8.5 MATHEMATICAL APPENDIX

8.5.1 Calculation of Dynamic Properties of Motor Proteins Using Derrida's Method

Here we present a detailed description of calculations of dynamic properties for linear sequential discrete-state stochastic models shown in Fig. 8.1. We follow closely the method originally developed by B. Derrida in 1983 (Derrida 1983) [40], which was later extended in different directions (Kolomeisky and Fisher 2007, Kolomeisky 2013) [84, 82].

Our starting point is the master equation for the temporal evolution of the probability function $P_j(l,t)$ to find the particle in the state j at the binding site l at time t,

$$\frac{dP_j(l,t)}{dt} = u_{j-1}P_{j-1}(l,t) + w_{j+1}P_{j+1}(l,t) - (u_j + w_j)P_j(l,t), \qquad (8.39)$$

which is identical to Eq. (8.3). Because of the periodicity, we have $N_{l-1} \equiv 0_l$, $u_j \equiv u_{j\pm N}$ and $w_j \equiv w_{j\pm N}$. Then the master equation for the border between two periods, $j = 0$, differs slightly,

$$\frac{dP_0(l,t)}{dt} = u_{N-1}P_{N-1}(l-1,t) + w_1 P_1(l,t) - (u_0 + w_0)P_0(l,t). \qquad (8.40)$$

It is convenient to define two new auxiliary functions for each state j,

$$B_j(t) \equiv \sum_{l=-\infty}^{+\infty} P_j(l,t), \quad C_j(t) \equiv \sum_{l=-\infty}^{+\infty} (j + Nl)P_j(l,t). \qquad (8.41)$$

The physical meaning of these functions can be explained in the following way. The function $B_j(t)$ gives a probability of finding the motor protein in the specific chemical state j independently of its position along the linear track. The function $C_j(t)$ corresponds to the average position of the motor when it is in the state j. The application of Eqs. (8.39) and (8.40) leads us to the following expressions describing the evolution of these new functions,

$$\frac{dB_j(t)}{dt} = u_{j-1}B_{j-1}(t) + w_{j+1}B_{j+1}(t) - (u_j + w_j)B_j(t), \qquad (8.42)$$

and

$$\frac{dC_j(t)}{dt} = u_{j-1}C_{j-1}(t) + w_{j+1}C_{j+1}(t) - (u_j + w_j)C_j(t) + u_{j-1}B_{j-1}(t)$$
$$-w_{j+1}B_{j+1}(t). \qquad (8.43)$$

We are interested in the dynamic behavior of the system in the stationary-state limit, i.e., when $t \to \infty$. At large times, we propose the following ansatz for these auxiliary functions,

$$B_j(t) \to b_j, \quad C_j(t) \to a_j t + T_j, \qquad (8.44)$$

where constant parameters b_j, a_j, and T_j can be determined from the dynamics of the system. These expressions are expected given the physical meaning of the functions $B_j(t)$ and $C_j(t)$. Note also that the periodicity implies

$$b_{j+N} = b_j, \quad a_{j+N} = a_j, \quad T_{j+N} = T_j. \qquad (8.45)$$

In the stationary-state limit we have $dB_j/dt = 0$, and from Eq. (8.42) we derive

$$w_{j+1}b_{j+1} - u_j b_j = w_j b_j - u_{j-1}b_{j-1}. \qquad (8.46)$$

One can introduce a function f_j,

$$f_j \equiv w_{j+1}b_{j+1} - u_j b_j, \qquad (8.47)$$

which is a probability flux between the states j and $j + 1$. At steady-state this flux is constant, $f_j = f_0$ for all j, and we can use this fact to determine explicitly the parameter b_j. By iteration we can write

$$b_j = -\frac{f_0}{u_j} + \frac{w_{j+1}}{u_j}b_{j+1} = -\frac{f_0}{u_j}\left[1 + \frac{w_{j+1}}{u_{j+1}}\right] + \frac{w_{j+1}w_{j+2}}{u_j u_{j+1}}b_{j+2} = \cdots. \qquad (8.48)$$

Continuing this procedure and taking into account that $b_{j+N} = b_j$, after $N-1$ steps we obtain

$$b_j = \frac{r_j}{R_N}, \quad r_j = \frac{1}{u_j}\left[1 + \sum_{k=1}^{N-1}\prod_{i=1}^{k}\frac{w_{i+j}}{u_{i+j}}\right], \qquad (8.49)$$

and $R_N = \sum_{j=0}^{N-1} r_j$.

To determine the coefficients a_j and T_j in Eq. (8.45) we employ Eq. (8.43), which leads to the following expressions,

$$w_{j+1}a_{j+1} - u_j a_j = w_j a_j - u_{j-1}a_{j-1}, \qquad (8.50)$$

and

$$a_j = [u_{j-1}T_j + w_{j+1}T_{j+1} - (u_j + w_j)T_j] + u_{j-1}b_{j-1} - w_{j+1}b_{j+1}. \qquad (8.51)$$

Comparing Eqs. (8.46) and (8.50) one might immediately conclude that

$$a_j = Ab_j, \tag{8.52}$$

where A is an unknown constant. Because of the normalization, $\sum_{j=0}^{N-1} b_j = 1$, we have

$$A = \sum_{j=0}^{N-1} a_j. \tag{8.53}$$

Summing up all Eqs. (8.50) and noting that all terms with T_j cancel out, yields

$$A = \sum_{j=0}^{N-1} (u_j - w_j) b_j. \tag{8.54}$$

Now using the expression for b_j, Eq. (8.48), we obtain

$$A = N \left[1 - \prod_{j=0}^{N-1} \frac{w_j}{u_j} \right]. \tag{8.55}$$

To get the function T_j requires more work. We introduce another auxiliary function,

$$y_j \equiv w_{j+1} T_{j+1} - u_j T_j. \tag{8.56}$$

Then Eq. (8.51) can be written as

$$y_j - y_{j-1} = a_j - u_{j-1} b_{j-1} + w_{j+1} b_{j+1}. \tag{8.57}$$

Since we now have the explicit expressions for a_j and b_j, these equations can be solved using the iteration procedure, similar to the one we used for finding b_j. It produces

$$y_j = u_j b_j + \frac{A}{N} \sum_{i=0}^{N-1} (i+1) b_{j+i+1} + c, \tag{8.58}$$

where c is an arbitrary constant. We will show later that the value of this constant is not important since it cancels out in the final expressions for dynamic properties. One can check that this expression solves Eq. (8.57) with the help of the relation

$$u_j b_j - w_{j+1} b_{j+1} = \frac{A}{N}. \tag{8.59}$$

The last equation can be understood if we use Eq. (8.54) and notice that the left side of Eq. (8.59) is the probability flux across the bond connecting the states j and $j+1$. In the stationary state it is the same for all bonds. Now we can return to Eq. (8.56), which can be iterated to obtain

$$T_j = -\frac{y_j}{u_j} + \frac{w_{j+1}}{u_j} T_{j+1} = -\frac{y_j}{u_j} - \frac{w_{j+1} y_{j+1}}{u_j u_{j+1}} + \frac{w_{j+1} w_{j+2}}{u_j u_{j+1}} T_{j+2} = \cdots . \tag{8.60}$$

Invoking the periodicity of the function T_j allows us to derive the expression

$$T_j = -\frac{1}{u_j}\left[y_j + \sum_{k=1}^{N-1} y_{j+k}\prod_{i=1}^{k}\frac{u_{i+j}}{w_{i+j}}\right] / \left(1 - \prod_{j=0}^{N-1}\frac{u_j}{w_j}\right). \tag{8.61}$$

Now we are fully prepared to calculate the velocity V and the diffusion constant D using definitions given in Eqs. (8.4) and (8.5). The average position of the motor protein in this model is given by

$$\langle x(t)\rangle = \frac{d}{N}\sum_{l=-\infty}^{+\infty}\sum_{j=0}^{N-1}(j+Nl)P_j(l,t) = \frac{d}{N}\sum_{j=0}^{N-1}C_j(t). \tag{8.62}$$

Using the master equation and the definition of the function $B_j(t)$ it can be shown that

$$\frac{d\langle x(t)\rangle}{dt} = \frac{d}{N}\sum_{j=0}^{N-1}(u_j - w_j)B_j(t). \tag{8.63}$$

At large times, it reduces to a simpler expression,

$$\frac{d\langle x(t)\rangle}{dt} = \frac{d}{N}\sum_{j=0}^{N-1}(u_j - w_j)b_j = \frac{d}{N}A. \tag{8.64}$$

Finally, the exact formula for the drift velocity is given by

$$V = \frac{d\left[1 - \prod_{j=0}^{N-1}\frac{w_j}{u_j}\right]}{R_N}. \tag{8.65}$$

One can easily find that for $N=1$ and $N=2$ the corresponding velocities are given by the expressions in Eqs. (8.6) and (8.7).

To obtain the explicit expression for the dispersion D we start from

$$\langle x^2(t)\rangle = \frac{d^2}{N^2}\sum_{l=-\infty}^{+\infty}\sum_{j=0}^{N-1}(j+Nl)^2 P_j(l,t). \tag{8.66}$$

Differentiating this equation and again using the master equation leads to

$$\frac{d\langle x^2(t)\rangle}{dt} = 2\frac{d^2}{N^2}\left[\sum_{j=0}^{N-1}(u_j - w_j)C_j(t) + \frac{1}{2}\sum_{j=0}^{N-1}(u_j + w_j)B_j(t)\right]. \tag{8.67}$$

Then utilizing the definition of the dispersion one can write

$$D = \frac{d^2}{N^2}\left[\sum_{j=0}^{N-1}(u_j - w_j)(a_j t + T_j) + \frac{1}{2}\sum_{j=0}^{N-1}(u_j + w_j)b_j - A\sum_{j=0}^{N-1}(a_j t + T_j)\right]. \tag{8.68}$$

It can be shown that terms proportional to t cancel out and we left with a simpler expression,

$$D = \frac{d^2}{N^2}\left[\sum_{j=0}^{N-1}(u_j - w_j)T_j + \frac{1}{2}\sum_{j=0}^{N-1}(u_j + w_j)b_j - A\sum_{j=0}^{N-1}T_j\right]. \qquad (8.69)$$

Finally, using expressions for the parameters T_j and b_j we obtain the explicit formula for the diffusion constant,

$$D = \frac{d}{N}\left[\frac{VS_N + dU_N}{R_N^2} - \frac{1}{2}(N+2)V\right], \qquad (8.70)$$

with

$$S_N = \sum_{j=0}^{N-1}s_j\sum_{k=0}^{N-1}(k+1)r_{k+j+1}, \quad U_N = \sum_{j=0}^{N-1}u_jr_js_j \qquad (8.71)$$

and a new function s_j defined as

$$s_j = \frac{1}{u_j}\left[1 + \sum_{k=1}^{N-1}\prod_{i=1}^{k}\frac{w_{j+1-i}}{u_{j-i}}\right]. \qquad (8.72)$$

One can show that for $N = 1$ and $N = 2$ the results from Eqs. (8.6) and (8.8) are recovered.

8.5.2 Calculation of First-Passage Probabilities and Dynamic Properties for $N = 2$ Linear Discrete-State Models

In this section we show how to compute the first-passage properties in the linear discrete-state model with $N = 2$. The problem is equivalent to the situation shown in Fig. 8.6. It is assumed that the molecular motor starts in the state 0, which corresponds to the binding site l along the linear track. We are interested in the statistics of reaching the state 2 (binding site $l + 1$) for the first time before reaching the state -2 (binding site $l - 1$). This can be found by analyzing the first-passage probability function $F_0(t)$. The temporal evolution of this distribution function is given by the corresponding backward master equation (see Fig. 8.6),

$$\frac{dF_0(t)}{dt} = u_0F_1(t) + w_0F_{-1}(t) - (u_0 + w_0)F_0(t), \qquad (8.73)$$

where $F_1(t)$ and $F_{-1}(t)$ are first-passage probability functions for starting in the position 1 or -1, respectively. For these functions the backward master equations are the following,

$$\frac{dF_1(t)}{dt} = u_1F_2(t) + w_1F_0(t) - (u_1 + w_1)F_1(t), \qquad (8.74)$$

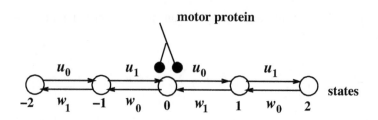

FIGURE 8.6 A schematic view for the discrete-state model with $N = 2$. The motor protein starts in the state 0, which corresponds to the binding site l. The state 2 describes the binding site $l + 1$, and the state -2 is identical to the binding site $l - 1$. The forward rates are u_0 and u_1, while the backward rates are given by w_0 and w_1.

$$\frac{dF_{-1}(t)}{dt} = u_1 F_0(t) + w_1 F_{-2}(t) - (u_1 + w_1)F_{-1}(t), \tag{8.75}$$

These equations can be solved via Laplace transformations. Then the backward master equations can be written as

$$(s + u_0 + w_0)\widetilde{F_0}(s) = u_0 \widetilde{F_1}(s) + w_0 \widetilde{F_{-1}}(s), \tag{8.76}$$

$$(s + u_1 + w_1)\widetilde{F_1}(s) = u_1 + w_1 \widetilde{F_0}(s), \tag{8.77}$$

$$(s + u_1 + w_1)\widetilde{F_{-1}}(s) = u_1 \widetilde{F_0}(s). \tag{8.78}$$

This system of equations can be easily solved, and we obtain

$$\widetilde{F_0}(s) = \frac{u_0 u_1}{(s + u_0 + w_0)(s + u_1 + w_1) - u_0 w_1 - u_1 w_0}. \tag{8.79}$$

All first-passage properties now can be explicitly evaluated. For the splitting probability of making forward step we have

$$\Pi_+ = \widetilde{F_0}(s = 0) = \frac{u_0 u_1}{u_0 u_1 + w_0 w_1}. \tag{8.80}$$

The mean dwell time to make the forward step is equal to

$$\tau_+ = -\frac{d\widetilde{F_0}}{ds}\Big|_{s=0} = \frac{u_0 + u_1 + w_0 + w_1}{u_0 u_1 + w_0 w_1}. \tag{8.81}$$

Similar calculations can be done if we want to evaluate the statistics of backward steps.

Collective Properties of Motor Proteins

9.1   COOPERATIVITY AND INTERACTIONS IN MOTOR PROTEINS DYNAMICS

Motor proteins are involved in a large number of biological processes. But their main functions, most probably, are to support different aspects of cellular transport as well as cellular processes that require exerting mechanical forces (Lodish et al. 2007, Alberts et al. 2007, Bray 2001, Howard 2001) [95, 4, 23, 68]. In this book, we already discussed various motor protein systems. Experimental and theoretical studies suggest that many motor proteins are strong enough as single particles to move rapidly and to exert large forces in biological cells. For example, kinesin motor proteins can be viewed as very efficient nanoscale machines that are able to perform individually multiple complex tasks (Howard 2001, Carter and Cross 2005, Clancy et al. 2011) [68, 27, 31]. Although single motor proteins can develop significant forces and run long distances along their tracks, many *in vivo* and *in vitro* experimental studies show that biological molecular motors usually work in groups (Ally et al. 2009, Holzbaur and Goldman 2010, Kulic et al. 2008, Soppina et al. 2008, Efremov et al. 2014) [6, 66, 90, 151, 47]. The number of motor proteins in these groups might vary. It is interesting to note that in many cases different types of motor proteins, even antagonistic to each other, might cooperate in performing their tasks.

    The fact that almost all motor proteins function in cells as teams is very surprising. We can understand the cooperativity of non-processive motor proteins (see Chapter 2) that can make only one or a few steps along their linear tracks before dissociating. The most famous example of such system is the muscles where non-processive myosins II work together to support its functioning (Howard 2001, Sweeney and Houdusse 2010) [68, 161]. Employing again the analogy between a cell and a large city, these biological molecular motors can be viewed as cars that carry together a very heavy load along the highway. But these machines frequently stall. They need to cooperate somehow with each other so that working machines keep moving the load while allowing the stalled cars to restart their engines. However, the situation is very different for processive motor proteins, such as kinesins, myosins V, myosins VI, dyneins, and many others, that individually can travel large distances along cellular filaments and can develop significant mechanical forces. These are very efficient machines that do not stall frequently. Still, many cellular cargoes are propelled by systems that include multiple copies of these motor proteins, and frequently these systems even involve molecular motors of different types.

These observations raise several important fundamental questions about motor proteins. Why do they cooperate? How does it happen at the molecular level? How do cells regulate the collective dynamics of motor proteins? Are some motor proteins more important than others for supporting cellular transport? Is this cooperativity always positive, i.e., leading to higher speeds, longer travel distances, and higher efficiencies for single motors working in groups? If not, what determines the sign of the cooperative interactions? How are collective properties of motor protein groups related to their single-molecule characteristics? How interactions specifically modify dynamic properties of motor proteins? Generally, the mechanisms of cooperativity in motor proteins are still not fully understood, and the impact of the collective dynamic behavior of molecular motors on various cellular processes is unclear. However, in recent years a clearer picture of these complex processes started to emerge due to significant advances in experimental and theoretical studies on cooperativity of motor proteins (Kolomeisky 2013, Driver et al. 2010, Driver et al. 2011, Uppulury et al. 2012, Uppulury et al. 2013, Efremov et al. 2014) [82, 45, 44, 170, 171, 47]. In this chapter, we will analyze the cooperativity processes in motor proteins using the physical-chemical concepts discussed in this book.

9.2 EXPERIMENTAL OBSERVATIONS

One of the main reasons that we still do not understand well the collective dynamics of motor proteins is that in *in vivo* experiments it is difficult to determine explicitly the nature, structures, and the precise number of molecular motors involved in the process (Driver et al. 2010, Driver et al. 2011, Kolomeisky 2013) [45, 44, 82]. In addition, it is frequently beyond the experimental capabilities to control these parameters reliably. Because of this, there are many controversial claims and observations on how teams of motor proteins might work together.

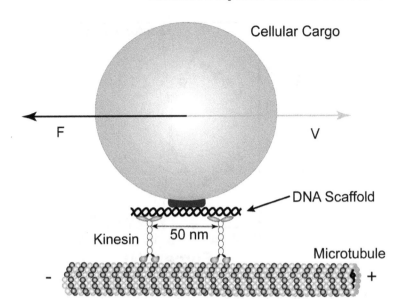

FIGURE 9.1 A schematic view of two kinesin motor proteins bound together in a complex via DNA scaffold. A protein complex transports a cellular cargo with a velocity V along the microtubule against the external force F. The size of the cargo is usually much larger (close to 1 μm) than shown in the figure.

These difficulties stimulated significant experimental efforts, and the breakthrough came with the development of the concept of synthetically made multi-motor complexes (Rogers et al. 2009, Furuta et al. 2013, Derr et al. 2012, Jamison et al. 2010, Ali et al. 2008, Lu et al. 2012, Rai et al. 2013) [134, 58, 39, 75, 5, 96, 129]. This is a very clever idea that utilizes the ability to investigate, with high precision, the dynamics of single particles. It was suggested to chemically couple several molecular motors by using proteins and/or DNA linkers (also called DNA molecular scaffolds). This is shown in Fig. 9.1 for two kinesin motor proteins that are coupled together in the complex. It is a non-trivial synthetic task since one has to be sure that the individual properties of motor proteins are not much affected. Then these complexes can be viewed as new "single molecules" that can be studied with all available single-molecule experimental tools. At the same time, motor proteins interact with each other, mimicking cooperativity in real cellular conditions. Furthermore, and most importantly, the nature and the number of biological molecular motors in these complexes are known exactly. This method provides a direct way to quantitatively test mechanisms of cooperativity for various motor protein systems (Kolomeisky 2013) [82].

The application of synthetically engineered complexes of motor proteins led to many surprising observations that underlined the differences in the collective dynamic properties of various classes of biological molecular motors.

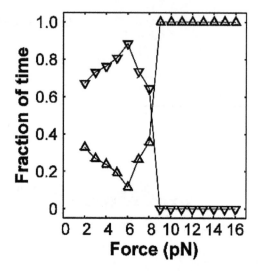

FIGURE 9.2   The fraction of time that the cellular cargo is moved by a single load-bearing motor (downward-pointing triangles) or by two load-bearing motors (upward-pointing triangles) at different external loads. The stall force for a single kinesin at these conditions is close to 8 pN. The figure is adapted with permission from Jamison et al. 2010 [75].

For assemblies of two coupled kinesin motor proteins that move the cargoes along the microtubules, optical-trap spectroscopic measurements indicated that these molecular motors cooperate negatively (Rogers et al. 2009, Jamison et al. 2010) [134, 75]. This means that two motors do not work together much, and most of the time the cargo is primarily translocated by only one of these motors. As shown in Fig. 9.2, experiments suggest that approximately 70–90% of the time (depending on the applied force) kinesin motors do not collaborate (Jamison et al. 2010) [75]. We call this cooperativity negative because the presence of one of the kinesins effectively knocks out the other one from active participation in the team. At the same time, a group of kinesin motor proteins sometimes was able to exert forces larger than the single motor could produce. In addition, two-motor complexes could also move faster than the single species. However, this collective dynamic behavior was rarely exhibited. Typically, when two kinesin motors were transporting the cargo against the external force, because of the geometry of binding (see Fig. 9.1), one of them (leading) was bearing most of the load (Jamison et al. 2010) [75]. This frequently led to the leading molecular motor's detachment from the microtubule filament. Increasing the number of motor proteins in the complexes did not change this collective behavior much (Furuta et al. 2013) [58]. These results strongly suggest that the intracellular transport depends quite weakly on the number of kinesin motor proteins. In other words, only a small number of kinesin motors actively participate in moving cellular cargoes.

This collective dynamic behavior of kinesins differs significantly from experimental results on other motor protein systems, such as Ncd (Furuta et al. 2013) [58] and myosins V (Lu et al. 2012) [96], where much more productive cooperation of biological molecular motors is observed. Individual Ncd motor proteins are non-processive, but the assembly of coupled molecular motors can run for distances exceeding 1 μm before detaching from the microtubule (Furuta et al. 2013) [58]. The run length also increased when the coupling between motors was stronger. This was done by decreasing the spacing between Ncd motor proteins connected to DNA segments. In contrast to kinesins, the force exerted by the team of Ncd motors increased linearly as a function of the number of proteins in the complex (Furuta et al. 2013) [58]. The collective dynamic properties of assemblies of multiple myosin V motor proteins are more complex, and they depend much more strongly (comparing with kinesins) on structural and mechanical properties of the system (Lu et al. 2012) [96]. But experiments also suggested that myosins V cooperate more productively than kinesins in the presence of temporary and spatially varying external loads (Lu et al. 2012) [96]. This was attributed to large step sizes and relatively small stall forces of single molecular motors.

Much more interesting behavior is observed when DNA origami scaffolds were utilized for coupling motors of opposite polarity (such as dyneins and kinesins) in one team to transport cellular cargoes (Derr et al. 2012, Diehl 2012) [39, 41]. The simplified view of this experimental system of antagonistic motor proteins is presented in Fig. 9.3. It was found that there are three possible dynamic outcomes depending on which group of molecular motors prevails. The cargo might be driven into the plus-end direction of the microtubule, which corresponds to kinesin motors dominating. In the case of dyneins winning, the cargo moves in the minus-end direction. There were also cases when the cargo could not move in either direction. This tug-of-war was a result of equal forces exerted by motors of opposite polarity. The motion can start only after one type of motor dissociates from the track (Derr et al. 2012, Diehl 2012) [39, 41]. Experiments show that dyneins tend to win this tug-of-war

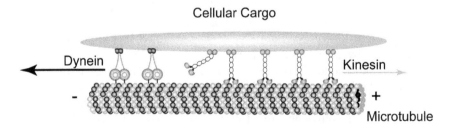

FIGURE 9.3   A schematic view of the tug-of-war phenomena in the bidirectional transport by two groups of motor proteins with opposite directionality. Dyneins try to push the cellular cargo in the direction of the minus-end on the microtubules, while kinesins try to move in the opposite direction.

more frequently. This observation is surprising because single dyneins generally exert lower forces than the single kinesins, as found by comparing the corresponding stall forces. But dyneins stay longer on microtubules and they cooperate positively, while only few kinesins participate in the tug-of-war and the overall cooperativity for them is rather negative, as was discussed above. The important conclusion from these experiments is that cellular transport can be regulated by tuning the number of dynein motor proteins while the effect of kinesins is much weaker.

Although the engineered multi-motor complexes were successful in clarifying many aspects of collective dynamics, one has to remember that their application is limited only to *in vitro* experimental systems. In addition, the fact that motor proteins in these complexes are chemically strongly coupled to molecular scaffolds might affect their dynamic properties in a way that is different from real cellular systems. Experimental *in vivo* studies with *quantitative control* on the number and properties of various types of motor proteins is still a challenge.

9.3   THEORETICAL IDEAS

Experimental studies of multi-motor complexes suggested that collective dynamics of motor proteins in cellular systems is very complex (Rogers et al. 2009, Furuta et al. 2013, Derr et al. 2012, Jamison et al. 2010, Ali et al. 2008, Lu et al. 2012, Rai et al. 2013) [134, 58, 39, 75, 5, 96, 129]. To some degree, we understand better now the basic features of individual molecular motors. But can it help us to explain cooperative phenomena exhibited by motor protein teams? This is the main theme of several theoretical methods proposed for analyzing collective properties of motor protein complexes (Klumpp and Lipowsky 2005, Campas et al. 2006, Driver et al. 2011, Uppulury et al. 2012, Uppulury et al. 2013, Muller et al. 2006, Kunwar and Mogilner 2010) [79, 26, 44, 170, 171, 116, 1]. It is interesting to note that all proposed ideas are based on discrete-state stochastic analysis of motor protein dynamics. In addition, only cytoskeleton transport phenomena were addressed.

The first proposed theoretical method postulated that in cellular transport each motor protein advances *independently of other molecular motors* (Klumpp and Lipowsky 2005) [79]. It was assumed that cellular cargoes are transported by groups of non-interacting motors that equally share the external loads and randomly bind and dissociate from the cytoskeleton filaments. In other words, each motor behaves like a single molecule that almost does not feel the presence of other motors in the team. The word "almost" is used here because the only effect due to other motors could be seen after the motor dissociation from the track when the external load was assumed to be quickly redistributed between motors that were still bound to the filament. This is a very simple and physically appealing theoretical picture that naturally couples single-molecule properties with dynamics of multi-motor complexes. It also allowed researchers to clarify some aspects of the tug-of-war phenomena (see Fig. 9.3) in the bidirectional transport by groups of motor proteins with opposite polarity (Muller et al. 2006) [116].

However, this approach had several weak points (Driver et al. 2010, Driver et al. 2011, Kolomeisky 2013) [45, 44, 82]. It assumed that most features of motor protein teams are additive, which essentially implies non-cooperative dynamic behavior. As a result, it is not possible to understand cooperativity phenomena in biological molecular motors using this approach. The method also utilized a linear force–velocity relations for single motors that is not very realistic. In addition, the description of binding/unbinding events was not thermodynamically consistent. Furthermore, the assumption of equal load sharing by motors was not justified from analysis of geometries of motor protein complexes. But most importantly, experiments do not agree with theoretical predictions from this approach (Rogers et al. 2009, Derr et al. 2012) [134, 39].

Analyzing the above theoretical method, one might conclude that its main problem is the neglect of interactions between motor proteins that work together. This stimulated a new theoretical approach that explicitly takes into account interactions of molecular motors with cargoes and with cellular tracks (Driver et al. 2010, Driver et al. 2011, Kolomeisky 2013) [45, 44, 82]. The main idea of this method is to enumerate the most relevant discrete states of the multi-motor system as shown in Fig. 9.4. These states differ by chemical conformations of each motor (bound or unbound) and by the distance between species attached to the cellular tracks. The utilization of single-molecule experimental measurements helps to calculate the total free energy of the system for each state. The detailed balance arguments are employed then to estimate the transition rates between different states, which is similar to the approach that was used for single motor proteins in the discrete-state stochastic models (Driver et al. 2010, Driver et al. 2011, Kolomeisky 2013) [45, 44, 82]. This provides a thermodynamically consistent description of all chemical transitions in the system. The temporal evolution of different states can be described by master equations, which are solved numerically exactly, providing a full dynamic description of the system (Driver et al. 2010, Driver et al. 2011, Kolomeisky 2013) [45, 44, 82]. It is a big advantage of the method that single-molecule chemical and mechanical data are used as input parameters for evaluating collective dynamic properties of motor proteins.

This theoretical method was tested in several *in vitro* experimental studies of engineered multi-motor complexes dynamics (Driver et al. 2011, Uppulury et al. 2012, Uppulury et al. 2013, Lu et al. 2012 [44, 170, 171, 96]. A good agreement with all observed experimental trends was found, underlining the importance of geometric and kinetic constraints in the mechanisms of the cooperative transport. The most important outcome of this method is the development of a microscopic picture of collective dynamics of motor proteins. It was argued that fast and efficient biological molecular motors, such as kinesins, do not like to collaborate during the cellular transport, leading to effectively negative cooperativity. At the same time, motor proteins that

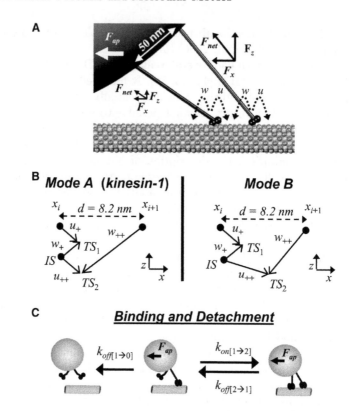

FIGURE 9.4   A discrete-state stochastic model for collective dynamics of multi-motor teams. (A) A schematic view of a two-kinesin complex. (B) Two variants of reaction coordinates for motor stepping along the filament. Mode A describes a situation when the forward transitions are not affected much by the load, and the velocity does not strongly depend on F. It corresponds to kinesins. Mode B describes the case when the forward transitions are affected by the load much more strongly. It corresponds to less-efficient processive motors. (C) Illustration of binding/unbinding chemical transitions in the system. The figure is reproduced with permission from Driver et al. 2011 [44].

are slow and not very efficient (e.g., dyneins and myosins V), with velocities decreasing rapidly under the effect of external loads, seem to collaborate more strongly. This is, clearly, a sign of positive cooperativity.

We can understand these microscopic arguments by comparing two typical force–velocity curves for motor proteins as illustrated in Fig. 9.5 (Kolomeisky 2013) [82]. In a team of motor proteins that jointly transport cellular cargo, the leading molecule experiences the largest fraction of the external load. In addition, the closer motors are to one another, the more they share the load. Let us analyze first the dynamics of two-kinesin assemblies. Kinesin motor proteins are strong, fast, and efficient, and their force–velocity relation

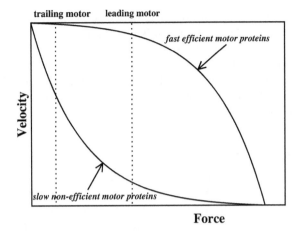

FIGURE 9.5 A schematic plot of typical force–velocity curves for individual motor proteins. The upper curve characterizes strong, fast, and efficient motor proteins like kinesins. The lower curve describes better weak, slow, and less-efficient motors like dyneins and myosins V. The vertical dotted lines correspond to forces and velocities experienced by leading and trailing particles in two-motor complexes.

is closely approximated by the upper curve in Fig. 9.5. We can see that for forces not close to the stall force, both leading and trailing motors have similar velocities. As a result, the trailing particle has a low probability of catching the leading motor. This means that most of the time kinesins do not share the load, and the largest force acts on the leading motor, forcing it to unbind from the cytoskeleton track more frequently. Recall that increasing the load on a motor protein also increases the probability of dissociation from the microtubule. This is a principal reason for the negative cooperativity observed in kinesin complexes. The situation is different for weaker, slower, and less-efficient motor proteins such as dyneins and myosins V. In this case, the lower curve in Fig. 9.5 better represents their force–velocity relations. Then for most loads the leading motor moves more slowly than the trailing motor, allowing it to keep it up with the leader. This leads to more load sharing by motor proteins and a lower probability for the leading motor to detach. Such dynamic behavior describes a positive cooperativity in multi-motor cellular transport.

Another crucial conclusion from this theoretical approach is the importance of the interaction strength between the motor protein and the cellular track for cooperativity. For very weak interactions, the collective dynamics is probably not very cooperative, while stronger interactions support more cooperative behavior. In application to real motor proteins, it was argued that the stronger cooperativity should be observed for dyneins and myosins V, while kinesins would prefer not to work together. This also implies that the regula-

tion of the cellular transport strongly depends on the number of dyneins and
myosins V, while the role of kinesin is less critical.

Despite significant advances in understanding the collective behavior of
motor proteins using the discrete-state stochastic approach with interactions,
the success is still quite limited. The main issue is that a fully quantitative
description is still not available. This is one of the most challenging problems
in the motor protein field.

9.4 SUMMARY

The important issue of the collective dynamics of multiple motor proteins
was discussed in this chapter. It was noticed that essentially for all cellular
processes, motor proteins function in groups. While this might be understand-
able for weak non-processive motors, the fact that even strong motors always
work in teams seems to be surprising. It was suggested that it is important
to understand the mechanisms of cooperativity in biological molecular motors
using physical-chemical concepts.

We then analyzed the experimental methods of studying collective dynamics of motor proteins. The earlier experimental attempts at investigating properties of multiple biological molecular motors were unsuccessful because the
quantitative information on the composition and chemical states of involved
motors was not available. Significant progress was achieved only after developing a method of artificially engineering multi-motor complexes by chemically
connecting individual molecules via DNA and protein scaffolds. This advance
led to several quantitative investigations of the dynamic behavior of multiple
motors. Using this experimental technique, it was shown that in multi-kinesin
assemblies, most of the time only one motor is active. This corresponds to
effectively negative cooperativity. A very different dynamic behavior is found
for complexes of several Ncd or myosin V motor proteins when the presence of
other molecules enhanced the dynamics of motors. This was an example of a
strong positive cooperativity. The method was later extended to teams of motor proteins that move in opposite directions along the cytoskeleton filaments,
dyneins, and kinesins. In this case, tug-of-war phenomena were observed. It
was found also that dyneins, despite being weaker motors, frequently win the
fight for the right to transport the cellular cargo over kinesins, which are
nominally stronger motors.

Then theoretical ideas of how to understand the collective dynamics of
motor proteins were discussed. The first proposed model assumed that motor
protein assemblies can be viewed as collections of independent single molecular
motors, whose properties we know quite well. This simple concept was powerful enough to explain several trends in multi-motor complexes. But it also had
several theoretical problems and experimental observation did not agree with
predictions from this approach. An alternative proposal was to extend the
original method for single motors to specifically include interactions between
motor proteins and cellular cargoes and cytoskeleton filaments. In addition, it

provided a thermodynamically consistent picture for all chemical transitions. This more advanced method was successfully utilized for analyzing several multi-motor systems. It also provided physical-chemical arguments concerning the microscopic origin of cooperativity in teams of biological molecular motors.

CHAPTER 10

Artificial Molecular Motors and Rotors

CONTENTS

10.1 INTRODUCTION

We have seen already in this book many examples that show the importance of motor proteins in supporting various cellular processes. Essentially, no biological systems can function without the involvement of motor proteins at different stages. As we discussed, the main reason for this is the ability of biological molecular motors to quickly and efficiently convert chemical, light, or thermal energy into useful mechanical work. Observations of high efficiency, strong power, flexibility, and robustness of these biological engines stimulated strong efforts to mimic them by developing similar synthetic nanoscale machines for various applications in sciences, medicine, and industry (Mavroidis et al. 2004, Shirai et al. 2006, Kay et al. 2007, Wang 2013, Abdelmohsen et al. 2014) [108, 147, 51, 179, 2].

Existing macroscale machines are much less efficient and less powerful (per unit mass) than biological molecules motors. Another important advantage of nanoscale-size machines is the ultimate control of any processes at the molecular level. This is one of the most important fundamental goals of science and technology! To approach this goal, a huge number of ideas on designing and creating artificial molecular motors were proposed (Kay et al. 2007, Wang 2013) [51, 179]. Significant synthetic successes have been achieved in many directions, opening routes for building real nanomotors (Mavroidis et al. 2004, Shirai et al. 2006, Kay et al. 2007, Wang 2013, Abdelmohsen et al. 2014) [108, 147, 51, 179, 2]. However, theoretical explanations of how these manmade nanoscale machines operate are still quite vague. One of the biggest mysteries in the field is to understand the collective behavior of synthetic molecular motors, i.e., the way they interact with each other when working in groups.

It is not possible to cover all these advances in the field of synthetic molecular motors in one chapter. It requires a full-volume book. Instead, we concentrate on several important trends and directions in developing artificial molecular machines, as well as on possible mechanisms of their functioning and their relations to biological motor proteins. Our approach again is based on the physical-chemical analysis of the underlying phenomena, which, as we showed in this book, seems to be very productive for understanding dynamic properties of molecular motors.

There are three main directions in which the development of synthetic molecular motors is proceeding. In one approach, the biological molecules (mostly DNA, RNA, and proteins), because of their unique chemical and mechanical properties, are utilized for creating the manmade nanosized machines of different types (Seeman 2005, Kay et al. 2007, Abdelmohsen et al. 2014) [144, 51, 2]. Another approach suggests employing the non-biological units that have simpler chemical structures, greater stability, and can be more easily controlled (Kay et al. 2007, Shirai et al. 2006, Wang 2013) [51, 147, 179]. A different direction describes multiple efforts to create artificial molecular rotors (Kottas et al. 2005, Lensen and Elemans 2012) [86, 92].

10.2   BIOLOGICAL ARTIFICIAL MOLECULAR MOTORS

The functioning of all biological systems is controlled by complex multimolecular complexes, consisting mainly of proteins and nucleic acid molecules, which can be viewed as nanoscale machines (Lodish et al. 2007, Alberts et al. 2007) [95, 4]. They actively work to maintain the cellular transport, cellular signaling, transfer of genetic information, and many other biological processes. It is clear that the excellent mechanical and chemical characteristics of these molecular machines are due to special properties of the individual molecules in the complexes. For this reason, researchers started to look into biological molecules as potential building blocks of artificial nanoscale machines (Yurke et al. 2000, Seeman 2005, Kay et al. 2007, Abdelmohsen et al. 2014) [185, 144, 51, 2].

For a variety of reasons, DNA molecules were chosen as the most promising candidates for constructing synthetic molecular motors (Yurke et al. 2000, Seeman 2005)[185, 144]. One of the main properties of DNA molecules, which allows them to serve so efficiently as genetic material, is their complementarity. This means that the two single-stranded DNA chains are very flexible, but they might combine together to make a much more rigid double-stranded segment if the chemical composition of each chain is *complementary* to each other. The concept of complementarity can be explained in the following way, which is shown schematically in Fig. 10.1. The DNA molecules are polymers that are made of 4 different types of nucleotide subunits known as adenines, cytosines, guanines, and thymins (Lodish et al. 2007, Alberts et al. 2007) [95, 4]. They are labeled as A, C, G, and T, respectively. Strong bonds between single-stranded DNA chains are created by pairing monomers A with T and G with C from different segments; see Fig. 10.1. This process is also called a *hybridization* and it leads to a rigid double-stranded DNA molecule. Two single-stranded DNA chains are complimentary to each other if each subunit on one chain can bind to the corresponding subunit on another chain (see Fig. 10.1). The complementarity provides a fundamental relation between the sequence and the structure of DNA. The double-stranded DNA segments could be easily dissociated back into two separate chains by moderate heating. The next important step was to realize that branched structures could be created from a partially complimentary single-stranded DNA pieces (Yurke et al. 2000, Seeman 2005)[185, 144]. This eventually led to creating multiple DNA structures with different geometry and topology, which were utilized for developing synthetic molecular machines (Seeman 2005)[144].

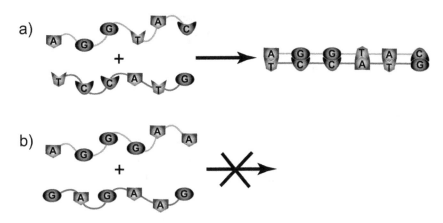

FIGURE 10.1   A schematic view of the complementarity between two DNA single-stranded segments. Hybridization takes place when A binds to T and G binds to C monomers. Geometric shapes of monomers reflect these observations. (a) Two single-stranded DNA chains are complimentary to each other because a perfect double-stranded segment can be formed. (b) Two single-stranded DNA chains that are not complimentary to each other.

To explain how the artificial machines made from DNA function, let us consider a specific example of the DNA molecular tweezers system (Yurke et al. 2000) [185]. This is illustrated in Fig. 10.2. The DNA-based molecular tweezers are prepared by mixing single strands labeled as A, B, and C (see Fig. 10.2a). Due to the complementarity, the chains B and C are able to bind to parts of the longer segment A to form rigid hands of the tweezers.

At the same time, the central part of A remains free and flexible so it can serve as a potential hinge for the tweezers hands motion. Two fluorescent dyes, specified as TET and TAMRA in Fig. 10.2, are attached to different ends of the segment A. They are used for monitoring the motion of the hands of the molecular tweezers, based on measuring the fluorescence intensity as a function of the distance between TET and TAMRA groups. If two dyes are close to each other, the fluorescence is quenched, lowering the signal. When two stiff arms of the tweezers are far away from each other, the fluorescent signal is strong, while the fluorescence decreases when they are close to each other. This is illustrated in Fig. 10.3.

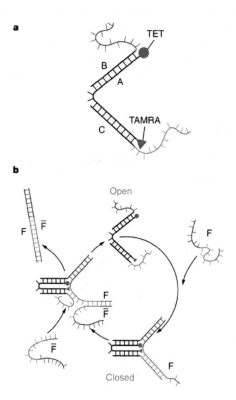

FIGURE 10.2 Creation and operation of the DNA-based molecular machine. (a) Schematic view of the structure of DNA molecular tweezers. The circle and triangle, labeled as TET and TAMRA, respectively, are fluorescent dyes. They are attached for monitoring opening and closing transitions. (b) Cyclic scheme of functioning DNA molecular tweezers. The closing starts after adding the DNA segment F, while opening proceeds with adding the complimentary DNA segment $\overline{F}$. The figure is adapted with permission from Yurke et al. 2000 [185].

The operation of this DNA-based molecular machine can be explained using Fig. 10.2b. It starts from the open configuration by adding a strand F, which has two regions that are complimentary to free parts of segments B and C. This hybridization reaction creates the closed conformation of the molecular machine by bringing two hands of the tweezers closer to each other. The thermodynamic driving force of this process is the formation of the double-strand bonds between F and the corresponding part of the molecular tweezers. To open the conformation, one needs to add the strand $\overline{F}$, which is fully complimentary to the strand F. It is important to note here that more chemical bonds are created during the hybridization at this stage because some part of the strand F was not hybridized in the previous step. This provides a favorable free-energy difference for the tweezers opening. The double-stranded segment $F\overline{F}$ is a waste product that must be removed from the system in order to maintain its operation. The free-energy difference for the molecular tweezers opening process can be written as

$$\Delta G = \Delta G_0 + RT \ln \frac{c(F\overline{F})}{c(\overline{F})}, \qquad (10.1)$$

where $c(F\overline{F})$ and $c(\overline{F})$ are concentrations of species $F\overline{F}$ and $\overline{F}$, respectively. As we discussed in this book, not removing the waste product would eventually shift the local equilibrium into the closed state and the molecular machine will not work. This is because the increase in the concentration of $F\overline{F}$ will make the free energy more positive, lowering the probability that the opening process might proceed.

The performance of this artificial DNA-based machine can be monitored by observing fluctuations in the fluorescence intensity as presented in Fig. 10.3. One can see that this motor is very slow; it takes approximately 1000 seconds to complete each cycle. Biological molecular motors, as we have seen already in this book, are much faster and can function for much longer periods of time. In addition, the molecular tweezers system is not *autonomous*. This means that in order to keep it working, one should constantly add and remove specific chemical compounds. This is another feature that makes this synthetic molecular machine less advantageous in comparison with real biological motors which can function on their own for long times. Furthermore, the interesting property of this system is that DNA was used both for constructing the motor as well as a fuel for its operation. To be more precise, the energy released during the hybridization processes was utilized for driving this artificial molecular engine. Similar ideas were also employed in more complex DNA nanomachines that were able to briefly proceed autonomously along one-dimensional tracks (Omabegho et al. 2009) [120]. However, even in this case the processivity and efficiency of these manmade nanoscale machines was quite low.

Synthetic molecular motors have also been developed using other types of biological molecules. One of the most interesting examples is a system known as *molecular spiders* (Pei et al. 2006, Lund et al. 2010) [124, 97]. They are

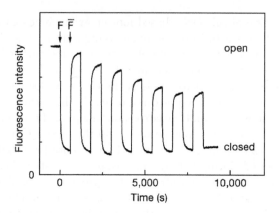

FIGURE 10.3 Fluorescent signal showing closing and opening of the DNA molecular tweezers after sequentially adding strands F and $\overline{F}$. The fluorescence peaks correspond to open configurations, while the lowest signals in fluorescence describe the closed forms of the molecular tweezers. The figure is adapted with permission from Yurke et al. 2000 [185].

shown in Fig. 10.4. Each spider consists of the main body made from a biological molecule streptavidin and several enzyme legs attached to it. Streptavidin is a protein molecule that is known to make very strong chemical bonds with some other biological molecules, and this property was employed in connecting enzymatic legs to the main body of the spider (Pei et al. 2006) [124]. Molecular spiders can proceed only along specific surfaces that are covered with nucleotides; see Fig. 10.4. Using their enzymatic legs, they catalyze the cleavage reactions in the nucleotides distributed on the surface (Fig. 10.4b). Since the interaction between the spider and the already catalyzed site on the surface is weaker than the interaction with uncatalyzed site, the molecular walker follows the path on the surface that finds nucleotides that are not catalyzed yet. This allows researchers to guide molecular spiders along specific prepared pathways, opening the exciting possibility for using them as molecular robots (Pei et al. 2006, Lund et al. 2010) [124, 97]. The energy gained during the enzymatic cleavage of double-stranded nucleotide segments is utilized by these molecular machines to move unidirectionally. It is important to note here that the motor must have several legs to keep it attached to the surface for long periods of time. These molecular spiders could walk distances up to 100 nm, but their speed was very low (≈ 3 nm/min) (Lund et al. 2010) [97]. In addition, their efficiency and power production were also much smaller than those of biological motor proteins (Lund et al. 2010) [97].

It is interesting to discuss the mechanism of the motion of molecular spiders since in many aspects it differs significantly from motor protein systems that we investigated so far. It was argued that molecular spiders follow the

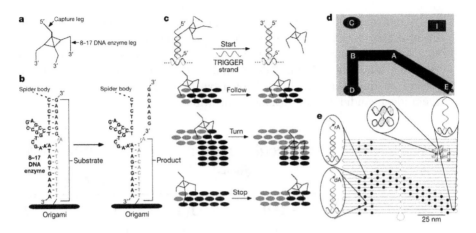

FIGURE 10.4 Synthetic biological molecular motors made of enzyme legs and a streptavidin core, called molecular spiders, that walk along specific surfaces by catalyzing attached nucleotides. (a) Schematic structure of the molecular spider. (b) Structure of nucleotides on the surface before and after the catalytic reaction with the spider. (c) The activity of the spider starts after dissociating from a single-stranded DNA segment. (d) A surface where the spiders can move. The dark region labeled EABD shows the part of the surface covered with nucleotides. E is a starting position, D is the final position. (e) More detailed representation of the molecular spiders walking along the surface. The figure is adapted with permission from Lund et al. 2010 [97].

so-called *burnt-bridge mechanism* (Antal and Krapivsky 2005, Artyomov et al. 2007) [7, 8]. To explain this let us consider a simplified one-dimensional picture of the process where the molecular spider is viewed as a single random walker on the lattice shown in Fig. 10.5. The molecular motor can hop with equal rates in both directions. But in contrast to previous random-walk models discussed in this book, the particle might interact with its linear track. For this reason, the lattice has three different types of the bonds; see Fig. 10.5. Strong links are not affected by the molecular motor. At the same time, weak links can be destroyed ("burned") with some probability when the particle moves through them from left to right. After the bridge is burnt, the motor is always on the right side of it. This is similar to the reaction of nucleotide cleavage catalyzed by molecular spiders on the surface. In addition, the motor cannot move back via the already destroyed bond. This leads to effective motion in the right direction. It corresponds to the experimental observation that molecular spiders cannot move along already catalyzed surface sites. This burnt-bridge mechanism explains the unidirectional motion and it also emphasizes the importance of the surface in driving and guiding these molecular machines. It is also important that theoretical calculations (Antal and Krapivsky 2005, Artyomov et al. 2007) [7, 8], in agreement with experimental observations (Lund et al. 2010) [97], suggest that molecular motors that follow the burnt-bridge mechanism are very slow, weak, and inefficient. But their functioning is fully autonomous and it is much more easily and precisely controlled than any other known synthetic molecular machines, making them ideal candidates for various applications.

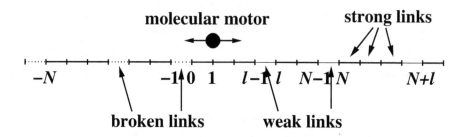

FIGURE 10.5 A schematic view of the burnt-bridge mechanism for molecular motors. The molecular motor is a random walker that hops with equal rates in both directions. The lattice has three types of sites. Thick solid lines correspond to strong links that cannot be burned. Thin solid lines describe weak links that can be destroyed when the motor crosses them from the left to the right. Already burned bridges are shown with dotted lines.

10.3   NON-BIOLOGICAL ARTIFICIAL MOLECULAR MOTORS

Although biological molecules possess superior chemical and mechanical properties for creating artificial nanoscale machines, they also have many limitations. The most important one is that thermal and chemical stability of these molecular complexes is quite low. For example, it is known that double-stranded DNA will melt at temperatures above 50–70 degrees Celsius, lowering the mechanical stability of DNA-built molecular machines at high temperatures. In addition, protein molecules become unfolded at high temperatures and in solutions of strong electrolytes (acids, bases, etc.). The denatured proteins have different mechanical properties, and their enzymatic ability is strongly reduced. This might limit the ability of manmade molecular machines to utilize enzymatic processes for fueling their motion. All these factors suggest that biological synthetic motors can work only in a very narrow range of conditions and they quickly degrade at more extreme situations. This might not be very useful for many technological applications.

There is a continued quest to develop microscopic machines that can be successfully utilized in various technologies at wider ranges of conditions. For this reason, there are multiple efforts in developing non-biological synthetic motors (Kay et al. 2007, Shirai et al. 2006) [51, 147]. A variety of physical and chemical ideas are being explored and in some directions a significant synthetic progress has been made. However, as we already mentioned, in most cases the mechanisms and functioning of these molecular motors are not well understood. Let us discuss several interesting examples of non-biological manmade nanoscale machines.

One of the most fascinating artificial motor systems is nanovehicles that move along metal surfaces (Shirai et al. 2006) [147]. They were created in 2005 when their wheel-assisted rolling motion along gold surfaces was demonstrated with the help of scanning tunneling microscopy (STM) methods. The first successful nanoscale machines are illustrated in Fig. 10.6. They are made from C_{60} (fullerene) molecules that are connected to other additional organic groups via complex multi-state chemical synthesis (Shirai et al. 2006) [147]. The four-wheeled complex is called a *nanocar*, while the three-wheeled machine is called a *nanotrimer*. It is interesting to discuss how the rolling motion of nanocars was proved in STM experiments (Shirai et al. 2006) [147]. In these experiments, the motion of nanocars and nanotrimers were monitored in parallel at 200 degrees Celsius. It was found that during the experiment nanotrimers did not move, while nanocars moved. The possibility of thermal hopping was neglected because nanotrimers did not show this. This observation led researchers to conclude that the translation was due to the rolling motion of the nanocars. The original fullerene wheels were later substituted with spherically symmetric carborane and Ruthenium-based complexes to create more efficient nanovehicles (Shirai et al. 2006) [147].

From a theoretical point of view, the microscopic origin of nanovehicles' dynamics is not well rationalized. It is clear that interactions between the wheels and the metal surface are critical for the motion. It is observed in experiments that the speed of nanocars on gold surfaces increases with temperature, indicating that the motion is thermally activated (Shirai et al. 2006) [147]. Extensive theoretical studies suggest that charge transfer and chemisorption play critical role in driving nanovehicles across metal surfaces (Akimov et al. 2012) [12], but explicit details are not fully worked out yet.

A different approach for developing artificial molecular motors is based on the idea of creating complexes that are engaged in asymmetric chemical reactivity (Howse et al. 2007, Kapral 2013) [69, 77]. This leads to different interactions between the molecule and the medium for different parts of the motor. As a result, the symmetry is broken and the motor is pushed in specific direction. This mechanism is called *diffusiophoresis*. This means that the particle moves due to the diffusion gradient created by the stronger chemical activity on one side of the molecule. It is illustrated in Fig. 10.7. The motor is viewed here as a spherical object where half of the surface is covered with specific chemical molecules that catalyze some chemical reactions. In these reactions more product molecules are produced than substrate molecules consumed, building a diffusion gradient in the system needed for the motion. As shown in Fig. 10.7, there are more molecules at the right side of the motor

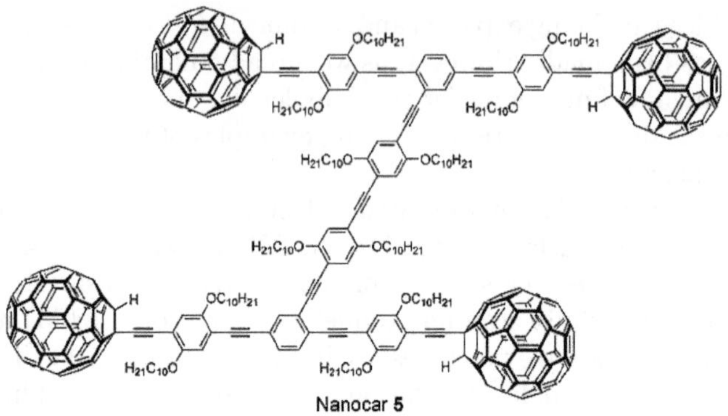

Nanocar 5

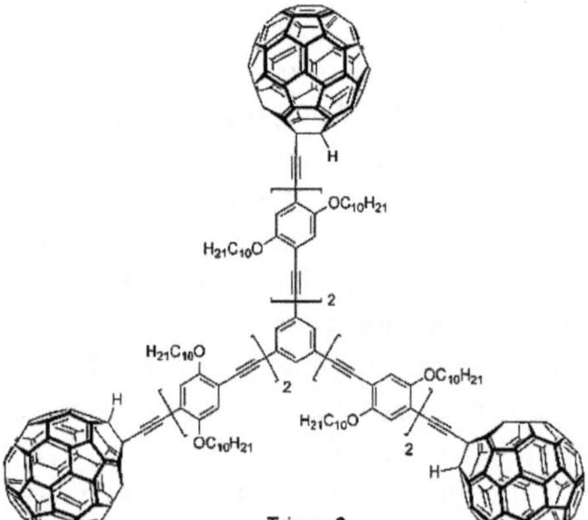

Trimer 6

FIGURE 10.6   Chemical structures of fullerene-based nanovehicles: the four-wheeled molecule is called nanocar, and the three-wheeled molecule is called a nanotrimer. The figure is adapted with permission from Shirai et al. 2006 [147].

than at the left side. This forces the motor to move to the left because there are more molecular collisions from the right side of the motor.

   This idea was realized in micron-sized polystyrene spheres where one side was coated with Pt (Howse et al. 2007, Kapral 2013) [69, 77]. These are known as *Janus* colloidal particles. The platinum atoms attached to the surface served to catalyze the reaction of hydrogen peroxide decomposition,

$$2H_2O_2 \leftrightarrow 2H_2O + O_2. \tag{10.2}$$

One can see that in this reaction from two molecules of peroxide three product molecules (water and oxygen) are created. Increasing the concentration of peroxide molecules forces the motor to move faster, reaching speeds on the order of microns per second (Howse et al. 2007) [69]! This is comparable to real motor proteins, but one should mention that the sizes of colloidal motors

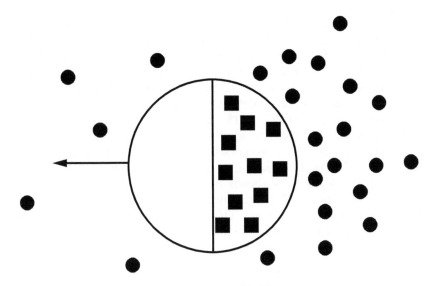

FIGURE 10.7 A schematic view of the molecular motor that is driven by diffu-siophoresis. Half of the surface of the motor is covered with molecules (filled squares) that catalyze the reaction of producing product molecules (filled circles). More product molecules are created on the right side of the sphere, which drives it to left (arrow).

are much larger. This is a very promising route to create artificial molecular machines. The only drawback of this approach is the relatively large size of the moving complex (in microns). It is desirable to have motors at the nanometer scale in order to influence phenomena at the molecular scale.

10.4 ARTIFICIAL MOLECULAR ROTORS

Molecular rotors form another important class of artificial molecular machines (Kottas et al. 2005, Lensen and Elemans 2012) [86, 92]. They are intensively studied because of many potential applications in science, medicine, and technology. Each molecular rotor usually consists of two parts: one of them is static and it is typically bound to some surface, while another part is mobile and it can rotate. There are many nanoscale rotating systems that were created and investigated using various synthetic methods (Kottas et al. 2005, Lensen and Elemans 2012) [86, 92]. In many aspects, molecular rotors behave similarly to translational molecular motors that we already discussed. Here we concentrate only on one example of such systems.

The rotation of dialkylsulfides (also known as thioethers) on Au(111) surfaces has been observed and investigated using STM experiments (Baber et al. 2008) [13]. Dialkylsulfides are made of a sulfur atom connected with two alkyl chains. To observe molecular rotations, thioethers are attached to the gold surface via the sulfur atom as shown in Fig. 10.8. It is known that sulfur makes strong bonds with gold atoms. Thus, in this case the sulfur atom is a stator, while the alkyl chains play the role of the rotor. STM measurements revealed that thioethers spin quite fast reaching speeds as high as 10^7 rotations per second (Baber et al. 2008) [13]. The experiments also indicate that the rotational motion of dialkylsulfides on gold surfaces is thermally activated: they spin faster at higher temperatures. These tests are done as described in Fig. 10.9. The rotating motion is viewed as hopping between several configurations where the rotor spends longer times. At these configurations the tunneling currents are different, which helps to identify those states and the hopping dynamics between them. This technique allows researchers to describe various aspects of rotational dynamics at different conditions.

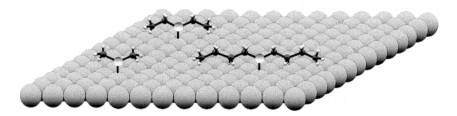

FIGURE 10.8   Thioethers on the Au(111) surface. Dimethyl, diethyl, and dibutyl sulfides are shown. The figure is adapted with permission from Baber et al. 2008 [13]. Copyright © 2008, American Chemical Society.

Theoretical investigations of surface-bound molecular rotors have revealed many surprising results (Kottas et al. 2005, Akimov and Kolomeisky 2011) [86, 11]. It was argued that the size and the symmetry of rotating chains, their flexibility, interactions with the surfaces, symmetry of the surfaces, and the chemical nature of the anchor groups are key elements that determine the dynamic properties of molecular rotors (Tierney et al. 2009, Akimov and Kolomeisky 2011) [163, 11]. For example, it was found in experiments that the rotational speeds of thioethers is independent of the length of the rotating arms for chains with two or more carbon atoms (Baber et al. 2008) [13]. This was a surprising observation since one could naively argue that increasing the length of the chains increases interactions with the surface, which should slow down the rotor. In other words, the friction should affect the rotational speed. Theoretical analysis using molecular dynamics computer simulations suggested that in this case the effect of compensation is taking place (Tierney et al. 2009, Akimov and Kolomeisky 2011) [163, 11]. Adding more atoms to the side branches does increase the interaction with the surface. At the same time, the steric repulsion between the alkyl groups and the gold surfaces increases the distance between anchor and the surface. This effectively leads to the

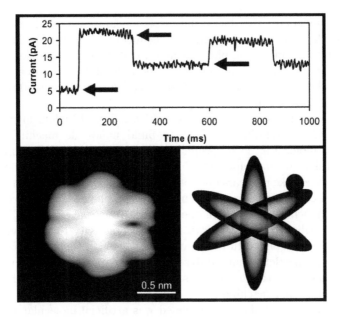

FIGURE 10.9   STM experimental measurements of rotational properties of di-alkylsulfides on Au(111) surfaces. The upper panel shows different tunneling current as a function of time due to hopping between different states. The lower-left panel shows the real image of rotational states for dibutyl sulfide. The lower-right panel presents a schematic view of possible rotational states for dibutyl sulfide. The figure is adapted with permission from Baber et al. 2008 [13]. Copyright © 2008, American Chemical Society.

lowering of the interaction per carbon atom, compensating for the effect of the length increase.

10.5   SUMMARY

In this chapter we discussed artificial molecular motors and rotors that were created as a way of developing miniature engines and devices. This development was also stimulated by attempts to mimic the properties of biological motor proteins. Many synthetic routes have been proposed and many mechanisms have been explored in the development of manmade nanoscale machines. It was argued, however, that theoretical understanding of artificial molecular motors is still quite limited for a variety of reasons. We identified three main directions of studies related to synthetic molecular motors.

The first approach is based on utilizing remarkable chemical and mechanical properties of biological molecules such as DNA, RNA, and proteins. We discussed the fact that the hybridization of DNA chains is a very convenient process for maintaining, controlling, and guiding synthetic molecular motors.

The mechanism of DNA-based nanoscale machines was analyzed on example of molecular tweezers using physical-chemical arguments. We later extended our analysis to more complex machines, called molecular spiders, that consist of various types of protein molecules. Possible theoretical mechanisms of molecular spider motion, based on so-called burnt-bridge ideas, were also extensively discussed.

The limited mechanical and chemical stability of biological synthetic motors stimulated significant efforts to build nanoscale machines from nonbiological molecules. Two specific systems and their mechanisms were discussed. First, we described the functioning of nanovehicles that roll along metal surfaces like real cars on roads. They consist of wheels that are made of fullerenes, carboranes, or ruthenium-based complexes. Various organic groups connect the wheels together in one complex. A second example discussed motors that utilized the asymmetric chemical reactivity to move via the diffusiophoresis mechanism. In these systems one side of the molecular machine is covered with particles that catalyze specific chemical reactions, creating diffusion gradient near the motor. This gradient is the main source of the motility of these molecular machines.

The last subject that we discussed was artificial molecular rotors. These complexes are made of two parts: one of them is static and the other one is rotating. The dynamics of molecular rotors is described using the example of thioethers spinning on gold surfaces. Theoretical ideas on important dynamic features of molecular rotors were also discussed.

CHAPTER 11

Future Directions in Studies of Motor Proteins and Molecular Motors

CONTENTS

11.1   WHAT WE UNDERSTAND NOW ABOUT MOTOR PROTEINS AND MOLECULAR MOTORS

Looking back into the topics discussed in this book, we realize now that our understanding of the motor proteins and molecular motors is more complete. This was accomplished mainly through huge progress in experimental and theoretical methods of investigation. But equally importantly, we found appropriate approaches for analyzing complex phenomena associated with motor proteins and molecular motors. The application of fundamental principles of physics and chemistry is the key to this success, and it allowed us to uncover many important features of these systems.

We learned first that motor proteins are biological molecules that participate in all major cellular processes. They support different mechanical and chemical aspects of biological organisms' functioning. Motor proteins can be viewed as nanoscale molecular machines that operate inside of biological cells. The main reason that they are so widely employed in cells is their unique abilities to transform chemical, light, or thermal energy into useful mechanical work. This work is needed for performing various biological functions. Another important feature of motor protein systems is the non-equilibrium nature of biological systems that allows molecular motors to reach very high efficiency, power and robustness during their work.

The development of single-molecule experimental methods opened the way for monitoring the activities of individual molecular motors with unprecedented spatial and temporal resolution. Molecular conformational changes in motor proteins have been observed with various experimental techniques, which gave a better view of how the transformation of energy into mechanical work is accomplished. Many experimental methods also provided a convenient way of modifying motor protein systems via application of external fields. Chemical kinetic and enzymatic studies helped us to understand where motor proteins take their fuel for actively working in biological cells. Motor proteins catalyze various chemical reactions and they utilize the energy released in these processes for supporting their mechanical activities.

Since the first discovery of motor proteins they have prompted significant discussions on the mechanisms of their functioning. Experimental successes in investigating biological molecular motors stimulated various theoretical ideas on mechanisms of molecular motors. We have discussed some them in detail in this book. These theoretical models allowed us to explain many observations on the dynamic properties of motor proteins, and provided a microscopic view of their activities. It was shown that the chemical transformations are strongly coupled with the production of mechanical forces in molecular motors. We can clearly state that we understand the main features of the dynamic behavior for most single motor proteins in *in vitro* conditions. Better understanding of motor proteins also assisted scientists in developing multiple artificial molecular motor systems that mimic the most useful properties of biological motors.

11.2   OPEN QUESTIONS AND PROBLEMS

Despite tremendous experimental and theoretical advances, our understanding of motor proteins remains incomplete. In order to continue our progress in explaining complex behavior of molecular motors, it is very important to clarify open issues and problems. Let us start by discussing several motor protein systems for which our knowledge of their dynamic behavior and microscopic mechanisms is still quite fuzzy. Currently, there are many motor proteins that are difficult to explain, and we can confidently predict that many new intriguing molecular motors will be discovered in the future. To be more specific, we concentrate on two motor protein systems that need better understanding at the molecular level.

Our first example concerns the bacterial flagellar motor (BFM), which is a rotary motor protein that we discussed in Chapter 2 (Berg 2003, Oster and Wang 2003, Sowa and Berry 2008, Mora et al. 2009) [18, 121, 152, 114]. The cryoscopic electron microscopy image of the rotary part of BFM is shown in Fig. 3.4, while the overall structure is given in Fig. 11.1. It is a very big multi-protein complex that sits in the bacterial membrane. BFM is one of the largest molecular machines operating in bacteria, with the overall molecular weight exceeding 1.1×10^7 grams per mole (Sowa and Berry 2008) [152]. The static part of the motor has a diameter close to 50 nm, and the long rotating filament attached to the base reaches a length of 10 microns. For comparison, the molecular weight of the kinesin motor protein, which is one of the most widely investigated motors, is close to 3.8×10^5 grams per mole, while its size in extended form is of order of 50 nm (Lodish et al. 2007, Vale 2003) [95, 172]. The BFM rotates long helical filaments with a speed reaching up to 100 rotations per second. Its motion is powered by electrochemical gradients created by fluxes of ions (H^+ or Na^+) across the bacterial membrane.

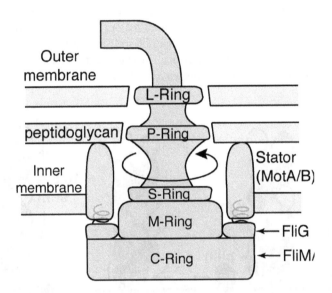

FIGURE 11.1   A schematic view of the main components of the bacterial flagellar motor. This motor is a multi-protein complex attached to the bacterial membrane. It controls the outside rotational motion of the filamentous extension, which is called a flagella. The figure is adapted with permission from Mora et al. 2009 [114].

The bacterial flagellar motor has been studied since the 1970s (Sowa and Berry 2008) [152]. However, the full picture of how rotations are generated at the molecular level is still not available. The main reasons for this are the following: (1) the very large size of this molecular motor; (2) very complex biochemistry associated with motor assembly, regulation, and functioning; and (3) the lack of high-quality structural data because the main part of macromolecular protein complex is bound to the membrane (Sowa and Berry 2008) [152]. Theoretical attempts to describe the complex dynamics of BFM have not been fully successful (Oster and Wang 2003,Mora et al. 2009) [121, 114]. It is very important to improve various aspects of experimental investigations of the bacterial flagellar motor, especially structural and biochemical, in order to build a comprehensive molecular picture of this motor protein complex. This should definitely lead to progress in the theoretical understanding of mechanisms in BFM.

Another interesting example of the motor protein systems that are not well understood is a protein complex known as type IV pilus (Maier et al. 2002, Maier et al. 2004, Burrows 2012, Craig et al. 2006) [103, 102, 25, 35]. It is shown in Figs. 11.2 and 11.3. Type IV pilus is a multi-component protein machine that consists of a base part attached to the bacterial membrane and thin (5–8 nm), long (up to several microns) filaments made of pilin proteins. The protein complex can stimulate the polymerization of these filaments, which extends their length, or depolymerization, which leads to retraction (Maier et al. 2002, Maier et al. 2004, Burrows 2012) [103, 102, 25]. It is coupled to ATP hydrolysis, although details are not well understood. Type IV pili play important roles in bacterial motility, in the creation of biofilms and in the transport of DNA and other species across the bacterial membrane.

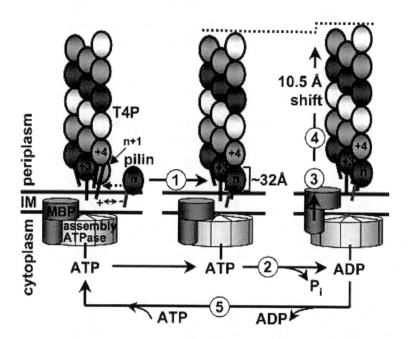

FIGURE 11.2   A schematic view of the type IV pilus motor protein complex and its functioning. The assembly of the pilin filaments, fueled by the ATP hydrolysis, is shown. The figure is adapted with permission from Craig et al. 2006 [35]

Experiments indicate that type IV pilus is one of the strongest motor proteins. The retraction of the pilin filaments in the single species can be stopped only by forces in the range of 100–150 pN (Maier et al. 2002, Maier et al. 2004) [103, 102]! With the help of type IV pili, bacterial cells can move consistently very large distances with speeds reaching several mm per hour (Burrows 2012) [25]. Experiments also suggest that multiple pili strongly cooperate with each other, but the details are still sketchy. Although some progress in studying type IV pilus molecular motors has been achieved, the number of open questions is significant. The structures of this protein machine are also poorly understood. It is not clear how the ATP hydrolysis is coupled with the force production. Why are the exerted forces so high? How is the transport of DNA and other species accomplished in pili? What is the mechanism of cooperativity? What is the role of the surface to which the type IV pili attach in driving the motility? It will be important to investigate these problems in detail to achieve a better understanding of the mechanisms of this biological molecular motor.

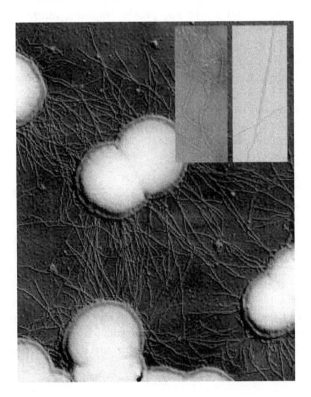

FIGURE 11.3 Scanning EM image of pili filaments coming out of bacteria. The clusters of bacteria cells are also created by the action of type IV pili motors. The figure is adapted with permission from Craig et al. 2006 [35].

In addition to specific motor proteins that are not yet understood, there are many general questions and problems for systems that are much better investigated. Although many features of motor proteins are still not determined, based on our discussions using fundamental concepts from physics and chemistry we can clearly say that we understand much better the dynamic properties of single molecular motors in *in vitro* conditions. However, the situation is not so bright when we think about the cases when many motor proteins work together. Despite some progress, the mechanisms of cooperativity in molecular motors remain obscured. To explain the complex dynamics of motor protein assemblies, many factors, including chemical and mechanical interactions and the effect of external forces, should be properly taken into account. One should also account for the highly dynamic nature of motor protein assemblies.

One of the most challenging tasks is to develop reliable experimental methods that would allow researchers to quantitatively measure the activity of motor proteins in real living cells. This will be an ultimate test for existing theoretical models, and it will also provide valuable information on how the functioning of motor proteins is coupled with other components of biological cells. There is also a big challenge for theoretical investigations of molecular motors. There is a significant gap in our understanding of structures of motor proteins and how they are related to their dynamic properties. The existing theoretical models for molecular motors are mostly phenomenological and coarse-grained, and the structural details are frequently neglected. It will be critically important to link various theoretical methods in order to develop a fully multi-scale description of biological molecular motors.

11.3 LOOKING INTO THE FUTURE

We have finished our journey in the fascinating world of motor proteins and molecular motors. Our road was not straight but it was full of surprising turns and observations. Our understanding of the field of motor proteins can be compared to a giant puzzle. We collected many individual pieces of this puzzle. Some of them we can even put together, while it is not clear how to connect others. But what is most important is that we have learned a strategy for assembling the pieces of the puzzle. The application of fundamental laws and concepts of physics and chemistry is our main guiding principle in analyzing biological molecular machines. Hopefully, this will help anyone who wishes to explore further the world of motor proteins and molecular motors.

Bibliography

[1] Kunwar A. and Mogilner A. Robust transport by multiple motors with nonlinear force-velocity relations and stochastic load sharing. *Phys. Biol.*, 7:016012, 2010.

[2] L.K.E.A. Abdelmohsen, F. Peng, Y. Tu, and D.A. Wilson. Micro- and nano-motors for biomedical applications. *J. Mater. Chem. B*, 2:2395–2408, 2014.

[3] A. Ajdari and J. Prost. Drift induced by a spatially periodic potential of low symmetry: pulsed dielectrophoresis. *C.R. Acad. Sci Paris*, 315:1635–1639, 1992.

[4] B. Alberts, A. Johnson, J. Lewis, M. Raff, K. Roberts, and P. Walter. *Molecular Biology of the Cell*. Garland Science, New York, NY, USA, 5th edition, 2007.

[5] M. Y. Ali, H. Lu, C.S. Bookwalter, D.M. Warshaw, and K.M. Trybus. Myosin V and Kinesin act as tethers to enhance each other's processivity. *Proc. Natl. Acad. Sci. USA*, 105:4691–4696, 2008.

[6] S. Ally, A.G. Larson, K. Barlan, S.E. Rice, and V.I. Gelfand. Opposite-polarity motors activate one another to trigger cargo transport in live cells. *J. Cell Biol.*, 187:1071–1082, 2009.

[7] T. Antal and P.L. Krapivsky. "Burnt-bridge" mechanism of molecular motor motion. *Phys. Rev. E*, 72:046104, 2005.

[8] M.N. Artyomov, A.Y. Morozov, E. Pronina, and A.B. Kolomeisky. Dynamic properties of molecular motors in burnt-bridge models. *J. Stat. Mech.*, page P08002, 2007.

[9] R.D. Astumian and M. Bier. Fluctuation driven ratchets: molecular motors. *Phys. Rev. Lett.*, 72:1766–1769, 1994.

[10] P. Atkins and J. de Paula. *Physical Chemistry*. W.H. Freeman New York, NY, USA, 9th edition, 2009.

[11] Akimov. A.V. and Kolomeisky A.B. Dynamics of single-molecule rotation on surfaces that depend on symmetry, interactions, and molecular size. *J. Phys. Chem. C*, 115:125–131, 2011.

[12] Akimov. A.V., C. Williams, and Kolomeisky A.B. Charge transfer and chemisorption of fullerene molecules on metal surfaces: application to dynamics of nanocars. *J. Phys. Chem. C*, 116:13816–13826, 2012.

[13] A.E. Baber, H.L. Tierney, and E.C.H. Sykes. A quantitative single-molecule study of thioether molecular rotors. *ACS Nano*, 2:2385–2391, 2008.

[14] J.E. Baker, E.B. Krementsova, G.G. Kennedy, A. Armstrong, K.M. Trybus, and D.M. Warshaw. Myosin V processivity: Multiple kinetic pathways for head-to-head coordination. *Proc. Natl. Acad. Sci. USA*, 101:5542–5546, 2004.

[15] I. Banga and A. Szent-Gyorgyi. Preparation and properties of myosin A and B. *Stud. Inst. Med. Chem. Univ. Szeged*, 1:5–15, 1942.

[16] T.E. Barman, S.R.W. Bellamy, H. Gutfreund, S.E. Halford, and C. Lionne. The identification of chemical intermediates in enzyme catalysis by the rapid quench-flow technique. *Cell. Mol. Life Sci.*, 63:2571–2583, 2006.

[17] D.A. Beard and H. Qian. *Chemical Biophysics. Quantitative Analysis of Cellular Systems.* Cambridge University Press, 2008.

[18] H.C. Berg. The rotary motor of bacterial flagella. *Ann. Rev. Biochem.*, 72:19–54, 2003.

[19] H.C. Berg. *Ecoli in Motion*. Springer Berlin, 2004.

[20] R.S. Berry, S.A. Rice, and J. Ross. *Chemical Kinetics and Dynamics.* New York: Oxford University Press, 2nd edition, 2002.

[21] P.D. Boyer. The ATP synthase—a splendid molecular machine. *Ann. Rev. Biochem.*, 66:717–749, 1997.

[22] S.T. Brady. A novel brain ATPase with properties expected for the fast axonal transport motor. *Nature*, 317:73–75, 1985.

[23] D. Bray. *Cell Movements: From Molecules to Motility.* Garland Publishing, New York, NY, USA, 2nd edition, 2001.

[24] G. Briggs and Haldane J. Die kinetik der unvertinwirkung. *Biochem. J.*, 19:338–339, 1925.

[25] L.L. Burrows. Pseudomonas aeruginosa twitching motility: Type IV pili in action. *Ann. Rev. Microbiol.*, 66:493–520, 2012.

[26] O. Campas, Y. Kafri, K.B. Zeldovich, J. Casademunt, and J.-F. Joanny. Collective dynamics of interacting molecular motors. *Phys. Rev. Lett.*, 97:038101, 2006.

[27] N.J. Carter and Cross R.A. Mechanics of kinesin step. *Nature*, 435:308–312, 2005.

[28] G. Charvin, D. Bensimon, and Croquette V. Single-molecule study of DNA unlinking by eukaryotic and prokaryotic type-II topoisomerases. *Proc. Natl. Acad. Sci. USA*, 100:9820–9825, 2003.

[29] Y. Chen. Asymmetry and external noise-induced free energy transduction. *Proc. Natl. Acad. Sci. USA*, 84:729–733, 1987.

[30] D. Chowdhury. Stochastic mechano-chemical kinetics of molecular motors: A Multidisciplinary enterprise from a physicist's perspective. *Phys. Rep.*, 529:1–197, 2013.

[31] B.E. Clancy, W.M. Behnke-Parks, J.O.L. Andreasson, S.S. Rosenfeld, and S.M. Block. A universal pathway for kinesin stepping. *Nature Struct. Mol. Biol*, 18:1020–1027, 2011.

[32] J.C. Cochran, J.E. Gatial, T.M. Kapoor, and S.P. Gilbert. Monastrol inhibition of the mytotic kinesin Eg5. *J. Biol. Chem.*, 280:12658–12667, 2005.

[33] P.F. Cook and W.W. Cleland. *Enzyme Kinetics and Mechanism*. Garland Science, New York, NY, USA, 2007.

[34] A. Cornish-Bowden. *Fundamentals of Enzyme Kinetics*. New York: Wiley-Blackwell, 4th edition, 2012.

[35] L. Craig, N. Volkmann, A.S. Arvai, M.E. Pique, M. Yeager, E.H. Egelman, and J.A. Tainer. Type IV pilus structure by cryo-electron microscopy and crystallography: Implications for pilus assembly and functions . *Mol. Cell*, 23:651–662, 2006.

[36] P. Cramer, D. Bushnell, and R. Kornberg. Structural basis of transcription: RNA polymerase II at 2.8 angstrom resolution. *Science*, 292:1863–1876, 2001.

[37] R.K. Das and A.B. Kolomeisky. Spatial fluctuations affect the dynamics of motor proteins. *J. Phys. Chem. B*, 112:11112–11121, 2008.

[38] E.M. De La Cruz and E.M. Ostap. Relating biochemistry and function in the myosin superfamily. *Curr. Opin. Cell Biol.*, 16:61–67, 2004.

[39] N.D. Derr, B.S. Goodman, R. Jungman, A.E. Leschziner, W.M. Shih, and S.L. Reck-Peterson. Tug-of-war in motor protein ensembles revealed with a programmable DNA origami scaffold. *Science*, 338:662–665, 2012.

[40] B. Derrida. Velocity and diffusion constant of a periodic one-dimensional hopping model. *J. Stat. Phys.*, 31:433–450, 1983.

[41] M.R. Diehl. Templating a molecular tug-of-war. *Science*, 338:626–627, 2012.

[42] K.A. Dietrich, C.V. Sindelar, P.D. Brewer, K.H. Downing, C.R. Cremo, and S.E. Rice. The kinesin-1 motor protein is regulated by a direct interaction of its heads and tail. *Proc. Natl. Acad. Sci. USA*, 105:8938–8943, 2008.

[43] M.S. Dillingham, Wigley D.B., and M.R. Webb. Direct measurement of single-stranded DNA translocation by PcrA helicase using the fluorescent base analogue 2-aminopurine. *Biochemistry*, 41:643–651, 2002.

[44] J.W. Driver, K.J. Jamison, K. Uppulury, A.R. Rogers, Kolomeisky A.B., and M.R. Diehl. Productive cooperation among processive motors depends inversely on their mechanochemical Efficiency. *Biophys. J.*, 101:386–395, 2011.

[45] J.W. Driver, A.R. Rogers, D.K. Jamison, R.K. Das, Kolomeisky A.B., and M.R. Diehl. Coupling between motor proteins determines dynamic behaviors of motor protein assemblies. *Phys. Chem. Chem. Phys.*, 12:10398–10405, 2010.

[46] D. Dulin, J. Lipfert, M.C. Moolman, and N.H. Dekker. Studying genomic processes at the single-molecule level: Introducing the tools and applications. *Nature Rev. Genet.*, 14:9–22, 2013.

[47] A.K. Efremov, A. Radhakrishnan, D.S. Tsao, C.S. Bookwalter, K.M. Trybus, and M.R. Diehl. Delineating cooperative responses of processive motors in living cells. *Proc. Natl. Acad. Sci. USA*, 111:E334–E343, 2014.

[48] A. Einstein. Uber die von der molekularkinetischen Theorie der Warme geforderte Bewegung von in ruhenden Flssigkeiten suspendierten Teilchen. *Annalen der Physik*, 322:549–560, 1905.

[49] C. Engel, S. Sainsbury, A.C. Cheung, D. Kostrewa, and P. Cramer. RNA polymerase I structure and transcription regulation. *Nature*, 502:650–655, 2013.

[50] V.A. Engelhardt and M.N. Lyubimova. Myosin and adenosine triphosphatase. *Nature*, 144:668–669, 1939.

[51] Kay. E.R., D.A. Leigh, and F. Zerbetto. Synthetic molecular motors and mechanical machines. *Angew. Chem. Int. Ed.*, 46:72–191, 2007.

[52] R.P. Feynman, R.B. Leighton, and M. Sands. *The Feynman Lectures on Physics*. Reading, MA: Addison-Wesley, 1966.

[53] J.T. Finer, R.M. Simmons, and Spudich J.A. Single myosin molecule mechanics: Piconewton forces and nanometer steps. *Nature*, 368:113–119, 1994.

[54] C.J. Fischer, L. Wooten, Tomko E.J., and T.M. Lohman. Kinetics of motor protein translocation on single stranded DNA. *Methods Mol. Biol.*, 587:45–56, 2010.

[55] M.E. Fisher and A.B. Kolomeisky. The force exerted by a molecular motor. *Proc. Natl. Acad. Sci. USA*, 96:6507–6602, 1999.

[56] K.A. Foster and S.R. Gilbert. Kinetic studies of dimeric Ncd: Evidence that Ncd is not processive. *Biochemistry*, 39:1784–1791, 2000.

[57] J. Frank. *Three-Dimensional Electron Microscopy of Macromolecular Assemblies*. Oxford University Press, New York, NY, USA, 2006.

[58] K. Furuta, A. Furuta, Y.Y. Toyoshima, M. Amino, K. Oiwa, and H. Kojima. Measuring collective transport by defined numbers of processive and nonprocessive kinesin motors. *Proc. Natl. Acad. Sci. USA*, 110:501–505, 2013.

[59] A. Gennerich and R.D. Vale. Walking the walk: How kinesin and dynein coordinate their steps. *Curr. Opin. Cell Biol.*, 21:59–67, 2009.

[60] I.R. Gibbons and A.J. Rowe. Dynein: A protein with adenosine triphosphatase activity from cilia. *Science*, 149:424–426, 1965.

[61] S.R. Gilbert and A.T. Mackey. Kinetics: a tool to study molecular motors. *Methods*, 22:337–354, 2000.

[62] A. Gnatt, P. Cramer, J. Fu, D. Bushnell, and R. Kornberg. Structural basis of transcription: An RNA polymerase II elongation complex at 3.3 A Resolution. *Science*, 292:1876–1882, 2001.

[63] W.J. Greenleaf, M.T. Woodside, and S.M. Block. High-resolution single-molecule measurements of biomolecular motion. *Ann. Rev. Biophys. Biomol. Struct.*, 36:171–190, 2007.

[64] D.D. Hackney. The tethered motor domain of a kinesin-microtubule complex catalyzes reversible synthesis of bound ATP. *Proc. Natl. Acad. Sci. USA*, 102:18338–18343, 2005.

[65] N. Hirokawa, Y. Noda, Y. Tanaka, and S. Niwa. Kinesin superfamily motor proteins and intracellular transport. *Nature Rev. Mol. Cell Biol.*, 10:682–696, 2009.

[66] E.L.F. Holzbaur and Y.E. Goldman. Coordination of molecular motors: From *in vitro* assays to intracellular dynamics. *Curr. Opin. Cell Biol.*, 22:4–13, 2010.

[67] P.L. Houston. *Chemical Kinetics and Reaction Dynamics*. McGraw-Hill, New York, NY, USA, 2001.

[68] J. Howard. *Mechanics of Motor Proteins and the Cytoskeleton*. Sinauer Associates Massachusetts, MA, USA, 2nd edition, 2001.

[69] J.R. Howse, R.A.L. Jones, A.J. Ryan, T. Gough, R. Vafabakhsh, and R. Golestanian. Self-motile colloidal particles: From directed propulsion to random walk. *Phys. Rev. Lett.*, 99:048102, 2007.

[70] J. Hurwitz, A. Bresler, and R. Diringer. The enzymic incorporation of ribonucleotides into polyribonucleotides and the effect of DNA. *Biochem. Biophys. Res. Commun.*, 3:15–18, 1960.

[71] A.F. Huxley. Muscle structure and theories of contraction. *Progr. Biophys. Biophys. Chem.*, 7:255–318, 1957.

[72] H.E. Huxley and J. Hanson. Changes in the cross-striations of muscle during contraction and stretch and their structural interpretation. *Nature*, 173:979–988, 1954.

[73] De Vlaminck I. and C. Dekker. Recent advances in magnetic tweezers. *Annu. Rev. Biophys.*, 41:453–472, 2012.

[74] H. Itoh, A. Takahashi, K. Adachi, H. Noji, R. Yasuda, M. Yoshida, and K. Kinosita. Mechanically driven ATP synthesis by F1-ATPase. *Nature*, 427:465–468, 2004.

[75] D.K. Jamison, J.W. Driver, A.R. Rogers, P.E. Constantinou, and M.R. Diehl. Two kinesins transport cargo primarily via the action of one motor: Implications for intracellular transport. *Biophys. J.*, 99:2967–2977, 2010.

[76] F. Julicher, A. Ajdari, and J. Prost. Modeling molecular motors. *Rev. Mod. Phys.*, 69:1269–1281, 1997.

[77] R. Kapral. Perspective: Nanomotors without moving parts that propel themselves in solution. *J. Chem. Phys.*, 138:020901, 2013.

[78] J.R. Kardon and R.L. Vale. Regulators of the cytoplasmic dynein motor. *Nat. Rev. Mol. Cell Biol.*, 10:854–865, 2009.

[79] S. Klumpp and R. Lipowsky. Cooperative cargo transport by several molecular motors. *Proc. Natl. Acad. Sci. USA*, 102:17284–17289, 2005.

[80] A.B. Kolomeisky. Exact results for parallel chains kinetic models of biological transport. *J. Chem. Phys.*, 115:7253–7259, 2001.

[81] A.B. Kolomeisky. Michaelis–Menten relations for complex enzymatic networks. *J. Chem. Phys.*, 134:155101, 2011.

[82] A.B. Kolomeisky. Motor proteins and molecular motors: How to operate machines at the nanoscale. *J Phys.: Condens. Matter*, 25:463101, 2013.

[83] A.B. Kolomeisky and M.E. Fisher. A simple kinetic model describes the processivity of myosin-V. *Biophys. J.*, 84:1642–1650, 2003.

[84] A.B. Kolomeisky and M.E. Fisher. Molecular motors: A theorist's perspective. *Ann. Rev. Phys. Chem.*, 58:675–695, 2007.

[85] A.B. Kolomeisky, E.B. Stukalin, and A.A. Popov. Understanding mechanochemical coupling in kinesins using first-passage time processes. *Phys. Rev. E*, 71:031902, 2005.

[86] G.S. Kottas, Clarke L.I., D. Horinek, and J. Michl. Artificial molecular rotors. *Chem. Rev.*, 105:1281–1376, 2005.

[87] Z. Koza. General relation between drift velocity and dispersion of a molecular motor. *Acta Phys. Polon.*, 33:1025–1030–450, 2002.

[88] F. Kozielski, S. Sack, A. Marx, M. Thormahlen, E. Schonbrunn, V. Biou, A. Thompson, E.-M Mandelkow, and Mandelkow E. The crystal structure of dimeric kinesin and implications for microtubule-dependent motility. *Cell*, 91:985–994, 1997.

[89] W. Kuhne. *Untersuchungen uber das Protoplasma und die Contractilitt.* Leipzig: Engelmann., 1864.

[90] I.M. Kulic, A.E.X. Brown, H. Kim, C. Kural, B. Blehm, P.R. Selvin, P.C. Nelson, and V.I. Gelfand. The role of microtubule movement in bidirectional organelle transport. *Proc. Natl. Acad. Sci. USA*, 105:10011–10016, 2008.

[91] A.W.C. Lau, D. Lacoste, and K. Mallick. Nonequilibrium fluctuations and mechanochemical couplings of a molecular motor. *Phys. Rev. Lett.*, 99:158102, 2007.

[92] D. Lensen and J.A.A.W. Elemans. Artificial molecular rotors and motors on surfaces: STM reveals and triggers. *Soft Matter*, 8:9053–9063, 2012.

[93] X. Li and A.B. Kolomeisky. Mechanisms and topology determination of complex chemical and biological network systems from first-passage theoretical approach. *J. Chem. Phys.*, 139:144106, 2013.

[94] J. Liu, D.W. Taylor, E.B. Krementsova, K.M. Trybus, and K.A. Taylor. Three-dimensional structure of the myosin V inhibited state by cryoelectron tomography. *Nature*, 442:208–211, 2006.

[95] H.A. Lodish, A. Berk, C.A. Kaiser, M. Krieger, M.P. Scott, A. Bretscher, H. Ploegh, and P. Matsudaira. *Molecular Cell Biology*. W.H. Freeman New York, NY, USA, 6th edition, 2007.

[96] H. Lu, A.K. Efremov, C.S. Bookwalter, E.B. Krementsova, J.W. Driver, K.M. Trybus, and M.R. Diehl. Collective dynamics of elastically coupled myosin V motors. *J. Biol. Chem.*, 287:27753–27761, 2012.

[97] K. Lund, A.J. Manzo, N. Dabby, N. Michelotti, A. Johnson-Buck, J. Nangreave, S. Taylor, R. Pei, M.N. Stojanovic, N.G. Walter, and E. Winfree. Molecular robots guided by prescriptive landscapes. *Nature*, 465:206–210, 2010.

[98] R.J. Lye, M.E. Poerter, Scholey, J.M., and J.R. McIntosh. Identification of a microtubule based cytoplasmic motor in the nematode *C. elegans*. *Cell*, 51:309–318, 1987.

[99] Nishiyama M., H. Higuchi, and T. Yanagida. Chemomechanical coupling of forward and backward steps of single kinesin molecules. *Nature Cell Biol.*, 4:790–797, 2002.

[100] Tomishige M., D.R. Klopfenstein, and R.D. Vale. Conversion of Unc104/KIF1A kinesin into a processive motor after dimerization. *Science*, 297:2263–2267, 2002.

[101] A.T. Mackey and S.P. Gilbert. Moving a microtubule may require two heads: a kinetic investigation of monomeric Ncd. *Biochemistry*, 39:1346–1355, 2000.

[102] B. Maier, M. Koomey, and M.P. Sheetz. A force-dependent switch reverses type IV pilus retraction. *Proc. Natl. Acad. Sci. USA*, 101:10961–10966, 2002.

[103] B. Maier, L. Potter, M. So, H.S. Seifert, and M.P. Sheetz. Single pilus motor forces exceed 100 pN. *Proc. Natl. Acad. Sci. USA*, 99:16012–16017, 2002.

[104] D.E. Makarov. Interplay of non-Markov and internal friction effects in the barrier crossing kinetics of biopolymers: Insights from analytically solvable model. *J. Chem. Phys.*, 138:014102, 2013.

[105] E. Mandelkow and E.-M. Mandelkow. Kinesin motors and disease. *Trends Cell Biol.*, 12:585–591, 2002.

[106] A. Marx, A. Hoenger, and Mandelkow E. Structures of kinesins motor proteins. *Cell Motil. Cytoskeleton*, 66:958–966, 2009.

[107] A. Marx, J. Muller, and Mandelkow E. The structure of microtubule motor proteins. *Adv. Protein Chem.*, 71:299–344, 2005.

[108] C. Mavroidis, A. Dubey, and M.L. Yarmush. Molecular machines. *Ann. Rev. Biomed. Eng.*, 6:363–395, 2004.

[109] A. Meglio, E. Praly, F. Ding, J.-F. Allemand, D. Bensimon, and Cro-quette V. Single DNA/protein studies with magnetic traps. *Curr. Opin. Struct. Biol.*, 19:615–622, 2009.

[110] A.D. Mehta, R.S. Rock, M. Rief, Spudich J.A., M.S. Mooseker, and R.E. Cheney. Myosin-V is a processive actin-based motor. *Nature*, 400:590–593, 1999.

[111] L. Meyer, D. Wildanger, R. Medda, A. Punge, S.O. Rizzoli, G. Donnert, and S.W. Hell. Dual-color STED microscopy at 30-nm focal-plane resolution. *Small*, 4:1095–1100, 2008.

[112] L. Michaelis and M. Menten. Die kinetik der unvertinwirkung. *Biochem. Z.*, 49:333–369, 1913.

[113] J.L.S. Milne, M.J. Borgnia, A. Bartesaghi, E.E.H. Tran, L.A. Earl, D.M. Schauder, J. Lengyel, J. Pierson, A. Patwardhan, and S. Subramaniam. Cryo-electron microscopy: A primer for the non-microscopist. *FEBS J.*, 280:28–45, 2013.

[114] T. Mora, H. Yu, Y. Sowa, and N.S. Wingreen. Steps in the bacterial flagellar motor. *PLOS Comp. Biol.*, 5:e1000540, 2009.

[115] S.P. Muench, Trinick J., and M.A. Harrison. Structural divergence of the rotary ATPases. *Q. Rev. Biophys.*, 44:311–356, 2011.

[116] M.J.I. Muller, S. Klumpp, and R. Lipowsky. Tug-of-war as a cooperative mechanism for bidirectional cargo transport by molecular motors. *Proc. Natl. Acad. Sci. USA*, 105:4609–4614, 2006.

[117] Golubeva N., A. Imparato, and L. Peliti. Efficiency of molecular machines with continuous phase space. *Europhys. Lett*, 97:60005, 2012.

[118] K.C. Neuman and A. Nagy. Single-molecule force spectroscopy: Optical tweezers, magnetic tweezers and atomic force microscopy. *Nature Methods*, 5:491–505, 2008.

[119] K.C. Neuman and A. Nagy. Video imaging of walking myosin V by high-speed atomic force microscopy. *Nature*, 468:72–76, 2010.

[120] T. Omabegho, R. Sha, and N.C. Seeman. A bipedal DNA Brownian motor with coordinated legs. *Science*, 324:67–71, 2009.

[121] G. Oster and H. Wang. Rotary protein motors. *Trends Cell Biol.*, 13:114–121, 2003.

[122] B.M. Paschal, H.S. Shpetner, and R.B. Vallee. MAP 1C is a microtubule-activated ATPases which translocates microtubules in vitro and has dynein-like properties. *J. Cell Biol.*, 105:1273–1282, 1987.

[123] A. Payen and J.-F. Persoz. Mechanisms and topology determination of complex chemical and biological network systems from first-passage theoretical approach. *Ann. Chim.*, 53:73–92, 1833.

[124] R. Pei, S.K. Taylor, D. Stefanovic, S. Rudchenko, T.E. Mitchell, and M.N. Stojanovic. Behavior of polycatalytic assemblies in a substrate-displaying matrix. *J. Aam. Chem. Soc.*, 128:12693–12699, 2006.

[125] T.D. Pollard and E.D. Korn. *Acanthamoeba* Myosin: I. Isolation from *Acanthamoeba Castelanii* of an enzyme similar to muscle myosin. *J. Biol. Chem.*, 248:4682–4690, 19733.

[126] A.M. Pyle. Translocation and unwinding mechanisms of RNA and DNA helicases. *Ann. Rev. Biophys.*, 37:317–336, 2008.

[127] H. Qian. Cycle kinetics, steady state thermodynamics and motors: A paradigm for living matter physics. *J. Phys.: Condens. Matter*, 17:S3783–S3794, 2005.

[128] Lipowsky R. and N. Jaster. Molecular motor cycles: From ratchets to networks. *J. Stat. Phys.*, 110:1141–1167, 2003.

[129] A.K. Rai, A. Rai, Ramaiya. A.J., R. Jha, and R. Mallik. Molecular adaptations allow dynein to generate large collective forces inside cells. *Cell*, 152:172–182, 2013.

[130] L. Reese, A. Melbinger, and E. Frey. Molecular mechanisms for microtubule length regulation by kinesin-8 and XMAP215 proteins. *Interface Focus*, 4:20140031, 2014.

[131] P. Reimann. Brownian motors: noisy transport far from equilibrium. *Phys. Rep.*, 361:57–265, 2002.

[132] S. Rice, A.W. Lin, D. Safer, C.L. Hart, N. Naber, B.O. Carragher, S.M. Cain, E. Pechatnikova, E.M. Wilson-Kubalek, M. Whittaker, E. Pate, R. Cooke, E.W. Taylor, R.A. Milligan, and R.D. Vale. A structural change in the kinesin motor protein that drives motility. *Nature*, 402:778–784, 1999.

[133] A.J. Roberts, T. Kon, P.J. Knight, K. Sutoh, and S.A. Burgess. Functions and mechanics of dynein motor proteins. *Nature Rev. Mol. Cell Biol.*, 14:713–726, 2013.

[134] A.R. Rogers, J.W. Driver, P.E. Constantinou, D.K. Jamison, and M.R. Diehl. Negative interference dominates collective transport of kinesins motors in the absence of load. *Phys. Chem. Chem. Phys.*, 11:4882–4889, 2009.

[135] Y. Rondelez, G. Tresset, T. Nakashima, Y. Kato-Yamada, H. Fujita, S. Takeuchi, and H. Noji. Highly-coupled ATP synthesis by F1-ATPase single molecules. *Nature*, 433:773–777, 2005.

[136] J. Rudnick and G. Gaspari. *Elements of the Random Walk*. Cambridge: Cambridge University Press, 2004.

[137] B. Rupp. *Biomolecular Crystallography: Principles, Practice and Application to Structural Biology*. Garland Science New York, NY, USA, 2009.

[138] Redner S. *A Guide to First-Passage Processes*. Cambridge: Cambridge University Press, 2001.

[139] Saka S. and S.O. Rizzoli. Super-resolution imaging prompts re-thinking of cell biology mechanisms. *Bioessays*, 34:386–395, 2012.

[140] Endow S.A. and Barker D.S. Processive and nonprocessive models of kinesin movement. *Ann. Rev. Physiol.*, 65:161–175, 2003.

[141] L. Schermelleh, R. Heintzmann, and H. Leonhardt. A guide to super-resolution fluorescence microscopy. *J. Cell Biol.*, 190:165–175, 2010.

[142] M.J. Schnitzer, K. Visscher, and S.M. Block. Single kinesin molecule studied with a molecular force clamp. *Nature Cell Biol.*, 2:718–723, 2000.

[143] J.M. Scholey, M.E. Porter, P.M. Grissom, and J.R. McIntosh. Identification of kinesin in sea urchin eggs, and evidence for its localization in the mitotic spindle. *Nature*, 318:483–486, 1985.

[144] N.C. Seeman. From genes to machines: DNA nanomechanical devices. *Trends Biochem. Sci.*, 30:119–125, 2005.

[145] U. Seifert. Efficiency of autonomous soft nanomachines at maximum power. *Phys. Rev. Lett*, 106:020601, 2011.

[146] J.R. Sellers and C. Veigel. Direct observation of the myosin-Va power stroke and its reversal. *Nature Struct. Mol. Biol*, 17:590–596, 2010.

[147] Y. Shirai, J.-F. Morin, T. Sasaki, J.M. Guerrero, and J.M. Tour. Recent progress on nanovehicles. *Chem. Soc. Rev.*, 35:1043–1055, 2006.

[148] M.R. Singleton, M.S. Dillingham, and D.B. Wigley. Structure and mechanism of helicases and nucleic acid translocases. *Ann. Rev. Biochem.*, 76:23–50, 2007.

[149] M. Smoluchowski. Zur kinetischen Theorie der Brownschen Molekularbewegung und der Suspensionen. *Annalen der Physik*, 326:756–780, 1906.

[150] G.A. Somorjai and Y. Li. *Introduction to Surface Chemistry and Catalysis*. New York: Wiley, 2nd edition, 2010.

[151] V. Soppina, A.K. Rai, A.J. Ramaia, P. Barak, and R. Mallik. Tug-of-war between dissimilar teams of microtubule motors regulates transport and fission of endosomes. *Proc. Natl. Acad. Sci. USA*, 106:19381–19386, 2008.

[152] Y. Sowa and R.M. Berry. Bacterial flagellar motor. *Q. Rev. Biophys.*, 41:103–132, 2008.

[153] J.A. Spudich, S.J. Kron, and M.P. Sheetz. Movement of myosin-coated beads on oriented filaments reconstituted from purified actin. *Nature*, 315:584–586, 1985.

[154] J.A. Spudich and S. Sivaramakrishnan. Myosin VI: An innovative motor that challenged the swinging lever arm hypothesis. *Nature Rev. Mol. Cell Biol.*, 11:128–137, 2010.

[155] J.I. Steinfeld, J.S. Francisco, and W.L. Hase. *Chemical Kinetics and Dynamics*. Upper Saddle River, New Jersey, Prentice Hall, 2nd edition, 1999.

[156] A. Stevens. Incorporation of the adenine ribonucleotide into RNA by cell fractions from *E. coli B. Biochem. Biophys. Res. Commun.*, 3:92–96, 1960.

[157] E.B. Stukalin and A.B. Kolomeisky. Transport of single molecules along the periodic parallel lattices with coupling. *J. Chem. Phys.*, 115:204901, 2006.

[158] H. Suzuki, K. Yonekura, and K. Namba. Structure of the rotor of the bacterial flagellar motor revealed by electron cryomicroscopy and single-particle image analysis. *J. Mol. Biol.*, 337:105–113, 2004.

[159] K. Svoboda and S.M. Block. Force and velocity measured for single kinesin molecules. *Cell*, 77:773–784, 1994.

[160] K. Svoboda, C.F. Schmidt, B.J. Schnapp, and S.M. Block. Force and velocity measured for single kinesin molecules. *Nature*, 365:721–727, 1993.

[161] H.L. Sweeney and A. Houdusse. Structural and functional insights into the myosin motor mechanism. *Ann. Rev. Biophys.*, 39:537–557, 2010.

[162] K. Thirumurugan, T. Sakamoto, J.A. Hammer, J.R. Sellers, and P.J. Knight. The cargo-binding domain regulates structure and activity of myosin 5. *Nature*, 442:212–215, 2006.

[163] H.L. Tierney, A.E. Baber, E.C.H. Sykes, Akimov. A.V., and Kolomeisky A.B. Dynamics of thioether molecular rotors: Effect of surface interactions and chain flexibility. *J. Phys. Chem. C*, 113:10913–10920, 2009.

[164] I. Tinoco, K. Sauer, J.C. Wang, and J.D. Puglisi. *Physical Chemistry. Principles and Applications in Biological Sciences.* Upper Saddle River, New Jersey: Prentice Hall, 4th edition, 2003.

[165] S. Toba, T.M. Watanabe, L. Yamagichi-Okimoto, Y.Y. Toyoshima, and H. Higuchi. Overlapping hand-over-hand mechanism of single molecular motility of cytoplasmic dynein. *Proc. Natl. Acad. USA Sci.*, 103:5741–5745, 2006.

[166] D. Toomre and J. Bewersdorf. A new wave of cellular imaging. *Annu. Rev. Cell Dev. Biol.*, 26:285–314, 2010.

[167] D. Tsygankov, M. Linden, and M.E. Fisher. Back-stepping, hidden substeps, and conditional dwell times in molecular motors. *Phys. Rev. E*, 75:021909, 2007.

[168] S.-R. Tzeng, M.-T. Pai, and C.G. Kalodimos. NMR studies of large protein systems. *Methods Mol. Biol.*, 831:133–140, 2012.

[169] S. Uemura, H. Higuchi, Olivares A.O., E.M. De La Cruz, and S. Ishiwata. Mechanochemical coupling of two substeps in a single myosin V motor. *Nature Struct. Mol. Biol.*, 9:877–883, 2004.

[170] K. Uppulury, A.K. Efremov, J.W. Driver, D.K. Jamison, M.R. Diehl, and A.B. Kolomeisky. How the interplay between mechanical and non-mechanical interactions affects multiple kinesin dynamics. *J. Phys. Chem. B*, 116:8846–8855, 2012.

[171] K. Uppulury, A.K. Efremov, J.W. Driver, D.K. Jamison, M.R. Diehl, and A.B. Kolomeisky. Analysis of cooperative behavior in multiple kinesins motor protein transport by varying structural and chemical properties. *Cell Mol. Bioeng.*, 6:38–47, 2013.

[172] R.D. Vale. The molecular motor toolbox for intracellular transport. *Cell*, 112:467–480, 2003.

[173] R.D. Vale, T.S. Reese, and M.P. Sheetz. Identification of a novel force-generating protein, kinesin, involved in microtubule-based motility. *Cell*, 42:39–50, 1985.

[174] van Kampen N.G. *Stochastic Processes in Physics and Chemistry.* Amsterdam: Elsevier, 2nd edition, 2001.

[175] C. Veigel and C.F. Schmidt. Moving into the cell: Single-molecule studies of molecular motors in complex environments. *Nat. Rev. Mol. Cell Biol.*, 12:163–176, 2011.

[176] G. Verley, K. Mallick, and D. Lacoste. Modified fluctuation-dissipation theorem for non-equilibrium steady states and applications to molecular motors. *Europhys. Lett.*, 93:10002, 2011.

[177] K. Visscher, M.J. Schnitzer, and S.M. Block. Single kinesin molecule studied with a molecular force clamp. *Nature*, 400:184–189, 1999.

[178] S. Walcott. The load dependence of rate constants. *J. Chem. Phys.*, 128:215101, 2008.

[179] D. Wang. *Nanomachines. Fundamentals and Applications*. Wiley-VCH, New York, NY, USA, 2013.

[180] T. Weidemann, J. Mucksch, and P. Schwille. Fluorescence fluctuation microscopy: A diversified arsenal of methods to investigate molecular dynamics inside cells. *Curr. Opin. Struct. Biol.*, 28:69–76, 2014.

[181] B. Widom. *Statistical Mechanics. A Concise Introduction for Chemists*. Cambridge University Press, Cambridge, UK, 2002.

[182] L.F. Wilhelmy. Ueber das Gesetz, nach welchem die Einwirkung der Sauren auf den Rohrzucker stattfindet (The law by which the action of acids on cane sugar occurs). *Annalen der Physik und Chemie*, 81:413–433, 1850.

[183] J. Xing, J. Liao, and G. Oster. Making ATP. *Proc. Natl. Acad. Sci. USA*, 102:16539–15646, 2005.

[184] A. Yildiz, J.N. Forkey, S.A. McKinney, T. Ha, Y.E. Goldman, and P.R. Selvin. Myosin V walks hand-over-hand: Single fluorophore imaging with 1.5-nm localization. *Science*, 300:2061–2065, 2003.

[185] B. Yurke, A.J. Turberfield, A.P. Mills, F.C. Simmel, and J.L. Neumann. A DNA-fuelled molecular machine made of DNA. *Nature*, 406:605–608, 2000.

Index

Milton Keynes UK
Ingram Content Group UK Ltd.
UKHW040100071024
449327UK00019B/682

9 780367 575762